The Wisdoms of
The Menopausal Godmother

EMMA GUY
Dip. Ac MATCM MAA RBAF

Embrace The Wisdoms

Emma x

What people are saying

ABOUT 'THE WISDOMS OF THE MENOPAUSAL GODMOTHER'

I got so much from this book, it's full of great advice and ideas. What's better still is that it's not just one voice talking about the menopause, from one angle. There are a wide range of women who bring their expertise to bear, from the worlds of nutrition, exercise and psychology. So, depending on how you're feeling or what your need is, you can pick and choose what supports you best. The book has also opened my eyes to different 'stuff' you can do to help ease your symptoms - I had no idea acupuncture could make an impact and I'm keen as mustard to try out THE GUY PROTOCOL.

Emma writes in a really upbeat and humorous style, bringing you along on the journey with good self-deprecating humour and insight of her own. It is of great comfort to know that so many women are experiencing middle life hormone changes in so many different ways.

Penny Haslam - Motivational Speaker &
Author of 'Make Yourself a Little Bit Famous'

Menopause! Hardly conjures up thoughts of youth, glamour and dare I say, sexy. No, when we think of the menopause, we think of sweaty women, shopping for fans and rubbing their HRT patch every time their partner looks at them sideways. And that's menopause in a nutshell. Or is it?

As a menopausal woman myself, after a nasty episode with breast cancer, I was chomping at the bit to read this book. How else could a book talk about us getting old, crabby and wondering when sex would be back on the menu? But Emma has written a book very different from the usual preaching of 'wear cotton', 'stop drinking', and 'curry is not your friend'. Emma's book opens a whole new world into alternative therapies to uneducated people like me. This book illustrates that coping with menopause is more than having a handy fan. With clear detail on how alternative therapies work, it gives women the confidence to explore these avenues from those who deliver them.

Emma's straightforward style will be appreciated by lots of women who don't know where to start when HRT isn't an option. Her contributors not only offer healing and supporting advice but also talk from experience without all of the 'menopausal hysteria'.

With many experts explaining how they can help, I have to say my favourite section is from the men who have lived or are still living with the menopause. This section made me realise just how much our partners experience and how 'invisibly' supportive they are.

THE WISDOMS OF THE MENOPAUSAL GODMOTHER is not about embracing old age. Thank God! This book is about embracing the new you. This book tells you that you are not on your own. This book tells you that we are all the same. This book tells you that you are still fabulous, will continue to be, and on your ropey days, there is so much you can do, besides HRT patches!

Estelle Maher - Author of 'The Killing of Tracey Titmass'

It's an honest story of strong belief and personal determination to offer hope, help & support to other women trying to navigate their way alone through the fog of menopause and its symptoms. The book is beautifully illustrated and the courage of her husband's account adds to its holistic approach and shows his love for Emma.

Wendy Wilson - Director of Care, St Luke's Hospice

This is an authentic and practically written book, sharing the author's extensive knowledge of acupuncture and evidence of a specific acupuncture protocol, developed by the author, to help menopause symptoms naturally. The book is very holistic and goes further to include easy to understand information about all the natural ways you can help yourself with managing your menopausal health and wellbeing. It is so easy to read and includes advice about nutrition, recipes, simple exercises, mindfulness, looking after your skin, hair and appearance and more. There is even a section for men and their perspectives! This book is going to help so many people. It is especially good for those of us who cannot take HRT, but all the advice and strategies are also very helpful to use alongside HRT.

Dr Annice Mukherjee - Top UK Hormone Specialist

Menopause mastery all in one place!!
THE MENOPAUSE GODMOTHER has "delivered" on her promise. Emma Guy has skilfully put together a book that caters for the complete newbie to all things menopause, acupuncture and holistic wellbeing. At the same time, she has provided a detailed and effective outline of her treatment THE GUY PROTOCOL for practicing acupuncturists who want to offer support to women going through the transition and, with her extensive network of therapists, Emma has created a place where you can window shop for other treatment options and experts available to help you with all stages of the menopause. I love the fact that Emma has included some testimonials from men here too. I am delighted to have been asked to contribute to this book and to witness the "birth" of the MENOPAUSAL GODMOTHER.

Dr Gill Barham - Menopause expert

Menopause can have debilitating effects for a woman. In this book, Emma, along with her tribe of other Godmothers, give practical tips that can be used at home, as well as guidance on how to find extra support. Acupuncture can have a profound effect on a person as it balances the whole body and THE GUY PROTOCOL speaks for itself in the number of women that it has helped.
Having the privilege of being part of a team that helps people live well with cancer, both with acupuncture and other lifestyle supportive tools, I have had the experience of seeing how people who go through changes, such as enforced menopause, can have their lives enhanced when troublesome symptoms are alleviated. This has a profound effect, not only on them, but on their families too. A protocol that helps women glide through the transition of menopause has the potential to affect many people's lives as we, as individuals, are not insular. When we treat the root cause, the effects ripple out

into the world. Emma sharing THE GUY PROTOCOL for other acupuncturists to use opens the door to help transform many millions of women's lives.

Amanda Reynolds – Health and Wellbeing Mentor.

THE MENOPAUSAL GODMOTHER is a must read for anyone going through the menopause or thinks they may be, but not sure. This book is full of useful information, hints and tips, including an explanation of what the menopause is and what symptoms to look out for and how to recognise them.

After going through chemotherapy, I was told I would probably start menopause in my 30- 40's. I have noticed in recent months changes to my physical and mental state resulting in me wondering (driving myself crazy!) whether or not I had started the menopause. After reading THE WISDOMS OF THE MENOPAUSAL GODMOTHER, I can now confirm at the lovely age of 39 (!) that I am perimenopausal. Thank you, Emma, for taking time to write such a fab book that will help and educate so many women. I will definitely be subscribing to the Facebook group and having a few of THE MENOPAUSAL GODMOTHER cocktails!

Sarah Pickles - Author of 'The Shock Factor'

Emma has written a book to help, guide, reassure and inspire women. She covers menopause and the role of alternative therapies, including acupuncture, in making this natural transition into a new phase of life. There are a lot of individual stories and personal recommendations from Emma and from others about gut health, lifestyle, exercise and more. Most women are going to find something new and useful to help them. But the strongest message that's coming across from the book is that you are not alone and that life is to be lived to the full as you embrace change and join the menopause club.

Jamie Hedger - The Healing & Acupuncture College

I particularly enjoyed the holistic approach and how THE WISDOMS OF THE MENOPAUSAL GODMOTHER pinpointed lots of different ways to help in the transition, with tasters that invited you to find out even more. The helpful links will be useful for any woman looking for ways to navigate the hormonal rollercoaster associated with menopause as well as women who are undergoing hormone-based treatment for breast cancer.

In essence, the book was interesting and very easy to read. Eye opening to me in relation to the acupuncture and full of helpful advice to women who are already on, or about to embark on the physical and emotional hormonal rollercoaster called the menopause.

Margo Cornish - Patron, Prevent Breast Cancer

Emma's candour is what gives her writing authenticity. It persuades you to root for her too.

THE WISDOMS OF THE MENOPAUSAL GODMOTHER is ambitious in its scope, not least in the range of perspectives and insight it provides, but it never stops short of being compelling. The value of acupuncture is an integral theme, although the reader is never preached to. Instead, the potential benefits to women from the practice – which have so transformed and enriched Emma's life both personally and professionally – serve only to make you want to know more.

Andrew Simpson - Freelance Journalist

The Wisdoms of
The Menopausal Godmother

EMMA GUY

The Wisdoms of The Menopausal Godmother
By Emma Guy

ISBN: 978-1-8384258-2-1

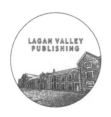

Printed by Lagan Valley Publishing

Cover Design by Gabriella Guy:
Millennial Burnout

Book design by Tanya Bäck,
www.tanyabackdesigns.com

Back Cover Photograph by Aga Mortlock,
www.agamortlockphotography.co.uk

Contents

Foreword

Have you started to write post-it notes with your kids' names on them? Do you need to change your underwear after every sneeze? Guess it's time to start gathering information on the menopause.

Menopause is one of those life changes. How we handle it is up to us. Whether we choose to use hormone therapy replacement, whether we set up our own physical and mental regime through exercise, diet, or other means, or whether we decide to "go it alone" and just ride it out until it's hopefully over, we are entirely responsible for the daily attitude we carry throughout this time.

The menopause often occurs at a time in our lives when most, if not all, of our children are leaving or have left the nest. (For some, it unfortunately happens when their off-spring are going through puberty which can cause fireworks.) We may begin to feel needed less. Our purpose in life seems to have left, along with its dirty washing and noisy music. It is a time when we might begin to question what lies ahead.

Now that we have more time to ourselves, we may begin to notice those indicators of age: facial wrinkles, the drooping turkey neck, and the triceps that are turning into the infamous "bingo wings". It's not a very appealing picture. However, we should not be concerned with the "old" woman who is staring at us in the mirror. We should concentrate on the "new" woman on the inside.

What can we do to get through this phase of our lives? Surprisingly there is much that we can do to stop blowing up at people and having a rough ride. We can take measures to look after ourselves and ensure we do not get too overwhelmed by what is happening to our bodies.

In *The Wisdoms of the Menopausal Godmother*, Emma Guy gives you the facts about the menopause – no fairytales. She has seen first-hand the benefits that acupuncture has on women and how it can transform the experience of the menopause.

Emma has also called on other Godmothers (including Yours Truly) to offer their advice on how to deal with the symptoms, and offer practical tips and advice which you won't find anywhere else.

So sit back, open a window if you are having a hot flush, and listen to what The Menopausal Godmother has to say.

And don't forget to laugh. In my opinion, the best medicine of all is laughter.

Question: What can a husband do when his wife is going through menopause?

Answer: Keep busy. If he's handy with tools, he can finish the basement. Then when he's finished, he'll have a place to live.

Carol Wyer

Carol is the author of award-winning comedies and best-selling crime novels. The DI Robyn Carter and DI Natalie Ward series have sold over half a million copies and been translated into several languages. She was the Winner of The People's Book Prize Award 2014/15. She was also responsible for one of the best books I've ever read on the menopause, 'The Grumpy Menopause'.

CHAPTER ONE

Where it all started

So who is The Menopausal Godmother? Well, let me introduce myself.

My name is Emma Guy, currently at the ripe age of fifty-one years old. I am married to Jonathan and have three children: Gabriella, Marcus and William. We live in Northwich, Cheshire, not far from the River Weaver.

At the moment I have many job roles – some would call me a "multiprenuer" – however, my transformation to becoming *The Menopausal Godmother* started in 2011 when I became a fully qualified acupuncturist. I then created my own business called *Acupuncture That Works* and opened a clinic not that far from where we live, just on the other side of the town.

Over the years, the business has grown from strength to strength. It is now a UK award-winning clinic with a team of therapists and practitioners offering a range of different disciplines.

> *A journey of a thousand miles begins with a single step.*
> Chinese Proverb

As I write this, I have over nine years' clinical experience, not only in my private clinic, but six years of that across two hospices as well. The realisation came to me suddenly – possibly after a glass of wine or two – that I have, over the years, treated thousands of women going through the menopause. Throughout this, I have helped them in with a wide range of debilitating symptoms which are part of their daily battle during this difficult life stage.

Consequently, I find myself in a position where I know a lot about the menopause, the symptoms, and the impact it can have on a woman's life.

You see, not only have I been helping women to deal with the diverse and incapacitating symptoms of menopause for nine years, but I also faced the trauma of an early menopause brought on by treatment for breast cancer at the age of 46. I remember one friend saying to me "how ironic that you treat so many breast cancer patients, and that you got it."

But little did I know that going through this dreadful period of my life would give me essential experience that would eventually become an advantage in helping so many others.

How I became an acupuncturist

It started back in 2006 after having William, my son – who is now, by the way, 15 years old and a proper teenager. Those of you who have children will know what that means! As long as he is fed and can sleep in most days (apart from school days) till midday, he is happy.

My pregnancy with William was quite good, with no major problems, no ongoing morning sickness and no sudden visits to the doctor. In fact, everything went really well, right up to the point when he was breech and I knew I was going to have to have a C-section. The birth didn't go to plan, as three attempts at a spinal block didn't work, so off I went to "La La land" under a general anaesthetic.

Waking up in the recovery room is something I will never forget, in both a bad way and a good way. In front of my eyes was Jonathan cradling William in his arms, a sight that turned me to tears because my little baby who I had carried all this time was healthy. The bad bit was that I couldn't feel my right leg. The feeling of joy became frightening. The midwives kept telling me that the feelings I had were normal and to get on with it. When I collapsed three days later it became clear to them that I had a Deep Vein Thrombosis (DVT) in my right leg, following which I was immediately put on Clexane injections. I'm not sure if you've ever had to inject yourself with anything, but let me tell you, this became an awful nightly ordeal, one which Jonathan could barely watch. I hated it and felt abandoned by the medical profession as there was no end in sight for this daily nightmare. Eventually, however, I complained to the doctors and, after expressing their surprise that I was still on them (no one had thought to provide a clear end date), they agreed that this torture should stop.

66

Menopause, the final frontier. These are the voyagers of women across the world.
To seek out new heights of stress, flushes and body changes. Where no man has gone before or would ever want to.
Phasers set to stun only, ladies, this could get messy!
HB

Shortly after this had finished, when William was four months old, I was diagnosed with ulcerative colitis. Certainly, the stress of the birth hadn't helped.

Over the following year I managed my ulcerative colitis with western drugs such as steroids but I still wasn't getting any better. When I look back now, every aspect of my life was very stressful at the time: the impact of William's birth, the subsequent injections, my stepfather was dying of cancer, I had a very stressful sales manager job and William was still dependent on me every day.

Sounds like a normal life for a woman, eh?

Working for Yellow Pages, managing a Field Sales team in Merseyside and South Manchester, was a high-pressure job. You were expected to not only achieve targets, but to overrun them.

I wanted to prove that, just like any other woman, I could do the consistent 12-hour days and work at weekends to catch up on paperwork. So, every morning I left the house around 07.30 and travelled to our offices – which were 15 miles away – to prove I was invincible. The job meant you were expected to hit the deck running and keep powering through to the end of the day, which could be as late as 9pm some nights. Not only was the job stressful, but I also had a family and household to look after. I'm sure some of this will sound familiar to many of you.

On one checkup for my ulcerative colitis my consultant suggested that I needed to take some time off as I was having a very bad flare-up at the time. In my usual "Supermum" mode, I thought, 'I'll have a couple of weeks off and then go back to work.' I wasn't one for taking time off work. I thought I would just take a little time off and get back to being Supermum quickly.

Unfortunately, two weeks turned into two months, which then turned into six months, and eventually twelve months. It seemed like once I had stopped, my body was getting worse and almost shutting down. I remember sitting on the sofa one afternoon (I hadn't washed and was still in my pyjamas), crying and rocking to myself. How could I be so ill? This was one of those moments when I wondered if I was ever going to get better.

Things could not continue the way they were, and after lots of research I decided to take a sabbatical from work and start a biomedicine course at Manchester University. Unfortunately, I couldn't continue with the course as was too poorly to even attend the lectures.

It was someone on this course, however, who suggested I tried acupuncture. My first thoughts were, "What on earth will that do for me? Surely it's all mumbo-jumbo, all modern day voodooism!"

With nothing to lose at that point though, I put aside my apprehensions and thought why not? I was on four different medications, including a delightful anal steroid foam. Oh, the joys of applying that every night was not only emotional but sometimes hilarious, as you can imagine.

So, I picked up the Yellow Pages and searched for "acupuncture" – even in 2009, this was still the best way to find local businesses as most of them had yet to get online.

With no expectations (and a head full of preconceived ideas), I went to see Rosie in October 2009. Rosie was a fully qualified acupuncturist and had been practicing for about ten years or so. She immediately made me feel at ease and started to ask me lots of questions about my overall health, habits and emotions, and much more. She also looked at my tongue and listened to my pulses. During that first session of acupuncture, I felt very relaxed and calm. After the first few sessions of acupuncture I started to feel a difference in my symptoms. How could this be? How or why was I starting to feel better? Surely it couldn't be acupuncture?

Five months later, in February 2010, I sat in my consultant's office and heard the impossible news that I had gone into remission with my ulcerative colitis. It was either a miracle or it was acupuncture. In my mind, I already knew the only thing I had changed, so it was at this point I fell in love with this ancient Eastern art.

I remember coming home after a session of acupuncture soon after this point and declaring to my husband, Jonathan, that I wanted to become an acupuncturist. The look of horror in his eyes as he nearly fell off his office chair will stay with me forever!

By not going back to work I would be forfeiting my AMG Mercedes, sick pay, holiday pay and a stable income. Jonathan, rightly, was concerned whether we would be able to cope with significantly less money coming into the household. Little did we both know that this was the start of an amazing journey.

Researching a suitable course turned out to be a lot more difficult than I thought. There were so many to choose from and, to be honest, most of them were two to three years of training, which I just couldn't commit to as they were so far away and I still had a young, now four-year-old, to look after.

However, after extensive searching, I finally found the perfect course at the Healing and Acupuncture College in Bath taught by Jamie Hedger. This was a condensed course over 12 months where you attended the college every other week for 3-4 days depending on the content you needed to cover. It was shorter but much more intense than the other courses I'd looked at and, as you can probably tell from my previous roles and behaviours, I was up for the challenge.

I have to say, it was hard being away from home every other week. However, the course suited me as there was no real downtime with studying. I was, in fact, continuously learning. Those who know me well know I get diverted very easily. In fact, it was always written in my school reports: "Emma could work harder if she wasn't easily distracted."

But despite this, a year later, after much hard work and commitment, I qualified as an acupuncturist. Woo Hoo! I could now officially stick pins in people and was proud to have letters after my name – Cert Ac. AHPR

It is funny how the universe sends you down a path. As luck would have it, Yellow Pages were looking to cut roles, so my boss and I came to an agreement and I left the business.

At this point I was qualified, but had no company name, nowhere to treat people and I was also missing one other ingredient – patients. So, what to call the business? After all, I was at this point because after all the pills Western medicine could throw at me, the only thing that worked was acupuncture. It wasn't a massive leap from there to the name, and so *Acupuncture That Works* was born.

Now I had a name and qualifications, but could I honestly run my own business and be successful at it?

I started on one day a week in the same room as Rosie, who if you remember was my acupuncturist. Although we never actually spoke about it directly, she became my mentor and someone I highly respected, someone I looked to for advice when I needed it.

Steadily, I built up my clinic from my first patient to then filling that one day a week. From there to three days a week was quite a slog, but within six months of grafting as hard as I could, I was up to full time.

Rosie, as always, helped me with advice when I needed it, and with her guidance, the clinic became a viable and thriving business. Keen to learn more, I continued my studies and added additional professional qualifications. Training at Shulan College in Manchester, I gained the next level up from Cert.Ac and become a Dip.Ac in 2013.

I was on a roll at this point and determined to increase my knowledge and understanding, so I trained and qualified in Tuina (Chinese Medical Massage) in 2013. I then started to explore the spiritual side a bit more, and over the next five years explored the world of Reiki, finally becoming a Reiki Master in 2019.

Fast forward to 2020 and I have been in business for nine years, run two clinics with seven other staff and treat between 30-50 patients a week. In 2019 we were awarded 'Global Health Pharma Acupuncture Clinic of the Year – UK' by the Alternative Medicine and Holistic Health Awards, which remains, to this day, my proudest moment in acupuncture. Now, far from just being an acupuncture clinic we are now seen as a health and wellbeing clinic, offering Physiotherapy, Reflexology, Reiki and Massage as well as Acupuncture, which still forms the core of the business.

Acupuncture inspired me in ways I had never felt before. It is a mission, a crusade, and once I was up and running, I was fascinated to see what the next adventure would be, where my acupuncture journey would take me.

The next step was quite unexpected, but then when fate is your guiding hand it can lead you anywhere.

Shaun, a fellow Parish Councillor at Lostock Gralam Parish Council, suggested I gained some experience after qualifying as an acupuncturist by volunteering my services at St Luke's Hospice in Winsford. Shaun had been having complementary therapy there after his operation for throat cancer.

So yet again, the great universe steered me there, as randomly, the following week, I was on a course in Crewe – and guess who I was sat next to? Pauline, the coordinator of all the complementary therapies at St Luke's Hospice. Fate was again guiding me.

Pauline is one of those people in life you meet for a reason. I now know that reason. She gave me the opportunity to shine as an acupuncturist. Pauline is the best boss I have ever had in my career. Why? Well, she is one of the good ones, always has your six[1] and I feel truly honoured to have her as a friend these days.

After volunteering at St Luke's Hospice for about a year

---

1 An American saying; to have someone's 'six' is equivalent to someone 'having your back' i.e. supporting you.

or so I noticed that most of my patients who were referred to the acupuncture clinic were sent there following breast cancer surgery. The main symptoms they presented were hot flushes, sleep disturbances and needing pain relief after their surgery. It was then I first saw a pattern emerging, so I experimented on acupuncture points.

The main objective was to get the hot flushes reduced, and in almost all the people I treated, it worked. Hot Flushes – or as I call them, "Tropical storms" (because not only do you get hot, you get a little bit of hurricane attitude – come on girls, we all know what I am talking about here!) – were a real issue for most of my patients. Getting some relief from these was a godsend for most of them.

After a few months of testing, I came up with the *Guy Protocol*, which was the combination of those acupuncture points that seemed to have the most positive impact on my patients' symptoms.

Looking back, it's clear now that this was the real birth of *The Menopausal Godmother*, as the discovery that acupuncture could help so many women in such a profound way paved the way for what was to come next. And what did come next was completely unexpected.

CHAPTER TWO

The Menopausal Godmother

Sometimes in our busy lives, all we need is to stop for a moment and think about what we want to do in the future. Like most people, I'd been too busy to stop until March 2020 when the Government announced that the entire country was locked down. The doors to my clinic closed immediately and, as things turned out, I didn't get to reopen again until July of that year.

Whilst the closing of the clinic was a real body blow, in hindsight it allowed me the one thing that I'd been denying myself for so long — time to think.

The concept of *The Menopausal Godmother* was born during this lockdown. It was during a brainstorming session on a Zoom call with Gill Barham that we first mentioned the idea. Gill was creating her own offering in this space of things menopausal, but the name didn't work with what she was planning to do. For me, however, it was like a million different ideas, suggestions and thoughts coalescing in a single moment around a name, a brand and an idea of how I could use my skills and experiences to help women around the world who are going through menopause. It was a moment of epiphany.

Everything that had gone before seemed to lead up to this moment. The years of acupuncture training and practice, my work in the hospice environment (specifically with patients suffering with hot flushes), and the growing number of women coming to see me for menopause-related symptoms — it all made sense.

On the back of this epiphany, I started a Facebook page – @menogodmum – back in September 2020 and launched my website – menopausalgodmother.co.uk – in mid-October. I definitely was not hanging around with this!

Since the Facebook page has gone live we have attracted hundreds of members and there are now over 1,000 posts, articles, ideas, questions, videos, interviews and fun items, all of which are there to support the members. I'm heartened by just how fast it's grown and it's down to the contributions of the members, who have taken it upon themselves to look after anyone who joins the group. If you need online support, I'd suggest you start there (see the graphic for details of how to join the Facebook group). The page is there for anyone suffering with (or needing information on) the menopause. It's regularly updated with information, fun facts and a dose of humour, which we all need at times.

There is also the Facebook group – *Menogodmum Members* – a private space in which members can share their issues and experiences and get help from other members and the other Godmothers.

The main point of this book is to give you knowledge about the menopause, to reassure you and to offer practical ways of dealing with it. As the *Menopausal Godmother*, I can not only give you advice on how to deal with the symptoms through acupuncture, but I can also share with you the accumulated knowledge gained over almost a decade of talking to women going through the menopause.

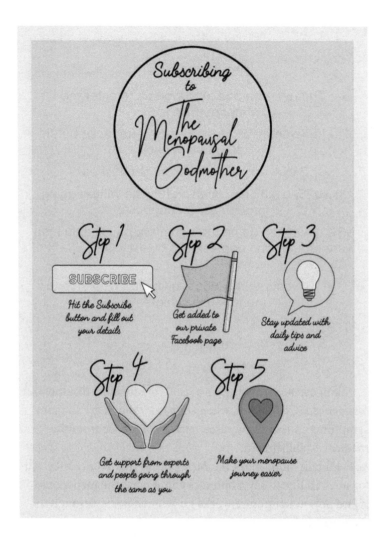

So, accepting that the menopause is something all women will go through (more of that later in the book), what are the key stats about the menopause that make it such a compelling subject for me?

DID YOU KNOW?

The average age for a woman to enter the menopause is 51.

1 in 100 women experience the menopause before 40 years of age.

3 in 4 women suffer from hot flushes.

In 2025, a billion women worldwide will be going through the menopause.

66% or women going through menopause said they were offered anti-depressants by their GP instead of HRT.

1 in 10 women think about giving up work due to menopause symptoms.

You can see why there is a need for someone like the *Menopausal Godmother*, when so many women get so many symptoms and, in some cases, such poor advice from the medical establishment.

I'll talk more about the *Menopausal Godmother* later, but for now, I'd like to say a bit more about what the menopause is and how acupuncture works for women going through the menopause.

CHAPTER THREE

The Menopause and Recognising The Symptoms

As a woman turning 50, I just hadn't seen it coming. Of course, some of the signs were already there, such as irregular periods, however I had missed or ignored them.

They call my menopause a surgical one. This means that literally overnight you could find yourself in the menopause, as opposed to a natural menopause which most women experience, where your oestrogen levels decline gradually over a period of time.

Prior to this point, I'd never given the menopause a second thought. Yes, I knew it existed and I also knew that it could affect women in different ways, but it was always something that happened to "other people". A bit like breast cancer, I suppose. I hadn't expected it to happen to me so soon.

So, as I say, when it started it came as a bit of a surprise.

At first, the symptoms were quite mild, something I could pass off without attributing it to the menopause or even giving them a name. But then they become more frequent and I got more of them. Waking up in the middle of the night in a hot sweat, sleep being disturbed, mood swings – all things you could put down to the weather or having a bad day. Individually, these weren't a problem, but when you start to group them together, it's a different matter. Some of these symptoms we now know to be called perimenopause (before menopause).

"

Duvet on, Duvet off!

SS

I suppose it started was when I was about 44 and my periods became erratic. Sometimes I would go three months without a period then have two in a month. Not only was this unusual when I'd been regular as clockwork for years, it was also inconvenient to say the least.

At the same time, I found that I started to experience odd hot flushes, sometimes in the daytime but most especially at night, where one minute I could be burning up and the next freezing cold.

Looking back, one of the other symptoms that I missed and failed to attribute to the menopause was panic attacks. There were a few occasions over the space of a couple of years where I simply became so panicked that I couldn't breathe. This was so unlike me. Normally confident and self-assured, to find that I was suddenly panicking over nothing was quite a fright.

Layer on top of this the occasional irrational behaviour and an intermittent grumbling backache and suddenly I was a different woman to the one I recognised as me.

"

I find cotton and linen clothes best as they are both warming and cooling and are less likely to make you sweat.

VP

30

And that's the problem. Any list of the symptoms of menopause will give you up to twenty different things that can present themselves. You may have read the list and thought "How on earth could anyone go through this and not spot that they are in menopause?" But the reality is that, like most problems in life, it's easier to look from the outside in than from the inside out.

As it turns out, the answer to how you fail to realise that you are in the throes of a major change in your life is quite simple. The symptoms don't happen all at once. It's a gradual accumulation of things which can easily be attributed to "getting older" or a general deterioration in health. And in between, you feel just fine. You feel your normal self, so surely "if I feel this good, I can't be going through the menopause?"

Wrong. It's a bitch and it creeps up on you with no warning, no fanfare and no chance to prepare you or your loved ones for it.

Of course, there are always exceptions, and some women have very few issues.

66

Thankfully I sailed through it with a positive mindset!
TM

What is the menopause?

There has been so much written about the menopause and what it is that there is little point repeating it here. However, I will give you an overview. At the back of the book I have listed a range of resources, some online and some in print, that you may find useful.

Generally, the menopause is typically defined as the point when a woman stops having periods and is no longer able to have children. Usually, women reach the stage when they are no longer able to get pregnant naturally between 45 and 55 years of age. The underlying reason for this is because a woman's oestrogen levels decline naturally as we age.

The word menopause – or as it was first noted, "*La menopause*" – was coined by French researchers in the early nineteenth century, and although there had been recognition of the condition since the seventeenth century, no one had formally researched and explored it.

Part of this is down to the fact that life expectancy and mortality rates in earlier centuries meant that women in particular were not expected to live into their fifties and therefore the number of people suffering symptoms was a relatively small group. Add to this the position of women in society, the state of general medical practice and the amount of interest people showed in the subject and you can understand why, even turning into the twentieth century, so little was known about the menopause.

We know where we get the word "menopause" from, but is it the correct name? Derived from Greek, menopause literally translates as "end of monthly cycles" and, because of this, it is often colloquially referred to as "The Change". Personally, I think that whilst "The Change" describes it well, it undersells what happens to a woman during this time. Frankly, I would like to rename it as "Oh shit, fucking bollocks, what is happening to me?" as that's a much better description of what really happens!

As women, we need to recognise that our hormones change and with that, so do our bodies. What we often fail to understand (possibly because this happens in such a relatively short space of time), is that it also affects how we look at our bodies. This is critical as the "self view" is so important in today's society. Women are often judged by the media and are affected by others' perception of how we should look, feel and act. Often underrated, this simple fact means that we go through huge amounts of unnecessary suffering as we see our bodies changing and find we are helpless to stop this happening.

> *It's like navigating a menopausal shit storm!*
>
> TT

Underlying all this is the simple fact that about half the population in the world will go through the menopause. Yes, read that sentence again! Half of the entire 7 billion population of the world – so around 3.5 billion people – will go through the menopause.

And is there a cure? Simple treatments that are universally applicable? Of course not. And that leads to a question I will cover later, which is "Why not?"

In the UK, the average age for going through the menopause is 51, but it varies in different parts of the world. A study by Thomas et al in 2001 found that across 26 countries (the age varied between 47 and 52), age at menopause seems to be mainly influenced by factors such as the reproductive history of individuals.[2]

On any day, week or month in the UK, about 13 million women are starting or finishing the menopause. That's almost 20% of the entire population of this country, but do you see it mentioned on the news bulletins every night?

Perhaps we should, as a staggering 60% of women will experience behavioural changes as well as the plethora of other symptoms. And yet we do not talk about it nearly enough.

But things are changing. Women are more likely to

---

2 https://www.jstor.org/stable/41465935

confide in each other and their partners. I am a member of two Facebook groups about menopause, each with over 9,000 women as members. That's got to be a good thing. And of course, as I've already mentioned, my own *Menopausal Godmother* private group, *Menogodmum Members*, is growing daily.

We try to get on with life whilst going through what can sometimes be debilitating symptoms.

As research for this book, I asked some friends, colleagues and patients for some feedback on menopause. Here is one that I particularly like and want to share with you all. I could not agree more.

Talk about it to your family and tell them what you are going through. They may not understand but at least they know how you are feeling.

SS

Perhaps this resonates with you? We may understand the symptoms of menopause and identify with them, but how often do we bury those feelings? Why do we? Perhaps it is because we have other things to consider, like work, family, cleaning, ironing, washing up etc. Here comes that "Supermum" mode again.

Another patient wrote:

Inconvenient – I was having a very nice life until it came along. When the hot flushes got too bad, I had to give up one of my jobs because I just could not function and I was having so many of them. I was lucky that I could afford to do that. I don't know how anyone could continue in that state. I think lack of energy is

34

something I have found hard to cope with too. I used to be much more active before and now find I just don't have the energy for a lot of tasks I used to do.

TT

What are the signs of the menopause?

I suppose it was the appearance of most of the "seven stages" all at once that finally convinced me I was going through the menopause. And on a day to day basis, I could cope with them, although some days it was harder than others.

When the realisation hit me, I could look back and see that these little buggers had been hounding my steps for the previous four years. Like little gremlins, they had been nipping at my heels for years but never all at the same time. Lots of little niggles, lots of annoying ailments, suddenly showing themselves to all be part of the same menopause onslaught.

Most women experience "seven stages of menopause", and just so you know what they are (for when they start coming after you), this little humorous list is the best I've found to describe them:

Itchy
Bitchy
Sweaty
Sleepy
Bloated
Forgetful
Psycho

Apart from the embarrassing hot flushes – which normally come in public at the most inopportune times – it's the mood swings that really get me. Even now, four years after I started the menopause, I still get them.

During a recent mood swing about nothing really,

Jonathan said to me, "I know this isn't you, it's the menopause" and it felt good that he had recognised it and was being so understanding – although it made me think, "Does he like me anymore?" You start to question every relationship when you are going through the menopause. At work, I just try and ignore the fact I am going through the menopause, primarily because I am so busy – which is a good thing. The impact, however, is felt more in the evening or the next day as I feel so fatigued. I read recently that up to 30% of women quit their jobs during their menopause as they just can't cope with the combination of symptoms and work pressures.

> 66
>
> *Mood swings mean it's like living with two different people.*
>
> JG

The hot flushes can be a real problem. Imagine a "flash in the pan" when you are cooking – you are at boiling point. This is what it is like to experience a hot flush. They come like waves. You so want to stop it, but you can't control them. Then the heat and sweat comes and this can last a few seconds or many minutes.

> 66
>
> *Wear layers so you can take some off when having a hot sweat.*
>
> AK

Personally, I particularly notice them more when I am drying my hair. Heat on heat. Sometimes after drying my hair, I have to walk around naked in the house to cool down. I have found that occasionally, at the last minute, I am forced to change plans for meeting up with friends as I simply can't cool down. It is the embarrassment of hot flushes and the strange anxiety that comes over you. But Jonathan doesn't seem to mind me strutting my stuff in my birthday suit!

Amongst the reams of literature about menopause, you can find list after list of the symptoms we can expect. It's like someone has simply opened a medical dictionary at random and picked out as many side effects as they can find. As far as I can see, the only thing missing is the warning not to operate heavy machinery, and given the mood swings I'm surprised that piece of advice isn't listed anywhere!

The lists of symptoms are endless, but if you spend some time on them, as I have, you will find that there are up to thirty-four different signs that you are going through the menopause.

SYMPTOMS OF THE MENOPAUSE

Hot flushes
Sleep disturbance
Mood swings
Irregular periods
Loss of libido
Vagina dryness
Fatigue
Weight issues
Forgetfulness
Depression
Incontinence
Backache
Headaches
Skin issues
Irritability

Are you experiencing any or all these symptoms? Do you feel normal? I know it doesn't make it any easier, but know you are not alone. As your *Menopausal Godmother*, I am also here to tell you that there IS something you can do about it.

Here are just a few suggestions from one of my patients:

"

1. Eat a healthy diet and try to lose weight if you need to. I've lost 2 1/2 stone and feel so much better for it. Avoid eating spicy food too late in the evening or that makes night sweats worse.

2. Take vitamin D for bone health

3. Plenty of moisturiser for skin dryness

4. Acupuncture!

MS

This advice leads me neatly into the role of acupuncture in helping with many of the symptoms. Knowing the massive impact these symptoms have on the lives of so many encouraged me to create the *Guy Protocol* of acupuncture. Before I explain the *Guy Protocol*, it is probably a good idea to tell you a little bit about acupuncture in general. If you are already familiar with acupuncture and how it works, then you can skip the next chapter.

CHAPTER FOUR

What is Acupuncture and How Does it Work?

You may already know all about acupuncture and what it can do. If so, please feel free to skip this chapter. For those of you who are not sure, or simply want a refresher on the basics, please read on.

In the interests of simplicity, I am going to try and keep this as clear as it can be. Far too often the descriptions of acupuncture make it sound like a dark art, but in practice it's quite straightforward.

Acupuncture is the process of inserting fine sterile needles, no thicker than a human hair, into a point along one of the "meridians" that run through your body. And in the spirit of keeping it simple, just accept that a meridian is a channel through which Qi (pronounced Chee) flows.

Even the word acupuncture says what it does on the tin. The word acupuncture has Latin roots, with "acus" meaning a needle and therefore "acupuncture" is to puncture with a needle.

No matter which history you choose to believe, acupuncture has been around for a very long time. Research suggests either that it was around in 6000BC, 3300BC or even

100BC.[3] Whichever you choose, it has roots that stretch back a long way. Contemporary records show that acupuncture has been practised continuously for over 3,000 years and, on that basis, can therefore be regarded as one of the most ancient practised forms of medical intervention known to man.

It is estimated that 2.3 million acupuncture treatments are carried out in the UK each year.

Acupuncture works on the principle that any pain or any illness is because your energy or your Qi has been disturbed in some way.

So, what is this Qi? Well, each cell in your body has adenosine triphosphate (ATP), an organic chemical that provides energy to drive living cells such as nerve impulses, muscle processes and chemical synthesis.

If you look at any medical diagram of the body at a cellular level, you can see that each energy cell is connected to another and from this arises the "connective tissue" in Western medicine. In Chinese medicine terms, however, this is the Qi. The Qi aligns along energy pathways called channels or meridians. As the *Menopausal Godmother*, my aim is to tap into these energy pathways and help to "reconnect" cells which may have stopped talking to each other.

So, what happens to the Qi or energy in the pathways?

Well, the Qi becomes blocked and therefore, acupuncturists needle into the acupuncture point to unblock the Qi and create a free flow of energy through the meridian. These channels or meridians are mostly called after the names of organs we all know and these are:
- Lung Channel
- Large Intestine Channel

3 https://academic.oup.com/rheumatology/article/43/5/662/1788282

- Stomach Channel
- Spleen Channel
- Heart Channel
- Small Intestine Channel
- Bladder Channel
- Kidney Channel
- Pericardium Channel
- Sanjiao Channel
- Gallbaldder Channel
- Liver Channel
- Du Channel
- Ren Channel

OK, so you may not have heard of Sanjao, Du and Ren, but all the rest are familiar? These channels go through different parts of the body, some running the entire length from head to toe, which explains why an acupuncturist may needle a point on your foot if you are suffering with headaches.

Of course, acupuncturists know what all these channels are and where they go, but just understanding that takes significant training. Much like a doctor going to university for seven years, acupuncture requires a thorough knowledge of the human body.

Their focus, however, is principally on the Qi, the energy that is in the meridian and how they can create some balance with acupuncture.

In Chinese medicine, the principle is that the energy lines along the meridians become blocked when there is any pain or illness. Acupuncture aims to remove blockages in the flow of Qi by diffusing lactic acid and carbon monoxide that accumulate in muscle tissue and can cause stiffness. These two culprits can also create abnormal pressure on nerves, lymph nodes and the blood vessels which often manifest in adversely affecting the function of the skeletal system and internal organs.

In my clinics, I often say to patients that Qi is like the M6 motorway and sometimes that motorway of energy becomes snarled up with traffic jams. If an acupuncture needle into a specific point along the meridian unblocks that jam, you would start to feel better.

Occasionally in clinic, a patient will have their first session of acupuncture and will notice an immediate difference, although most patients tend to report significant change after their third or fourth session. In this respect, acupuncture is little different to Western medicine in that it is not an immediate "cure" for anything. Typically, if you are prescribed tablets for any kind of illness you are told to take the whole course and, over time, you will hopefully see your symptoms reduce. Similarly, a course of acupuncture is recommended because it takes time to realign the Qi in the body and get it flowing correctly again.

Which brings us to the question, "Why does the Qi get blocked?"

Broadly speaking, energy or Qi blockages in Chinese medicine terms can be divided into internal blockages and external blockages.

External blockages are, as the name suggests, things that happen outside of your body. They could be based on the weather (hot or cold), or a break, fall or operation, or even something environmental that has happened to you, such as being exposed to chemicals.

Internal blockages are all about the seven basic emotions:

- joy,
- grief,
- sadness,
- fear,

- anger,
- stress and
- worry.

What we tend to see in most of our patients is a mixture of both internal and external blockages. The starting point for any acupuncturist will be to find out what your causable factor or factors are, as in a lot of cases there will be more than one thing blocking your energy. When you go for your first acupuncture session, therefore, don't be surprised if you are asked a lot of questions about what has happened in your life, either recently, or in some cases as far back as childhood. If you can be honest with your acupuncturist you may be very surprised at how effective acupuncture can be for restoring physical and emotional balance.

As you might expect, the Chinese have a proverb for this:

"

Everything comes from the mind.

This is so important as a great many patients we see are deeply affected by something that has happened in their past, and in many cases they have simply buried the memory. But the mind never forgets and its mere presence in the memory can be enough to cause a blockage in the Qi.

What this means is that acupuncture can (and is) used to treat an enormous range of complaints. Sometimes people present with a bad back or sore shoulder, but this could be related to an earlier problem. So whilst acupuncture is probably best recognised as a treatment for a range of pain issues, it can also be used for so many other things, from fertility to Achilles heel, from persistent verrucas to dry eyes. There really is no end to what acupuncture can do!

What to expect in your first session of acupuncture

On your first session of Traditional Chinese Medicine (TCM) acupuncture, you will have a Full Traditional Chinese Medicine consultation which will include some questions about you overall wellbeing.

As I mentioned, you may even be asked about your childhood or when you first started your periods as this information is essential for getting to the root cause and therefore knowing which meridian and points to needle. Typically, this in-depth consultation will also include a tongue and pulse diagnosis, at the end of which you will be given a Chinese Medicine diagnosis.

You should also be given an idea of what your treatment plan looks like and how many sessions you will need. This is important, as acupuncture is akin to muscle memory and I often say to patients you don't go to the gym for one session and get a perfect body. (If only, eh!) It takes time to train the Qi and for your energy to become much more balanced.

Once you get that balance then you need regular "top ups" to remind the Qi to be balanced. Just like having have your hair done, it's all about the maintenance and feeling good.

I can notice when I need a top up of acupuncture as my hot flushes start to come back.

AK

How does it work?

In modern day society, most people just want to know two things:

Does it work?

How does it work?

…and this is usually followed by "fix me!"

You really don't need to know the ins and outs of everything we learn over 2-3 years as Traditional Chinese Medicine Acupuncturists. However, we do like to educate you a little at each session of acupuncture. There is no point in you going home and your partner asking "So, what did they do?" if the only answer you can give is "they stuck pins in me". Understanding is not essential, but it helps, so we like to give you a little education to help you to firstly understand which points we have used, and secondly (and probably more importantly), why.

The physical process of acupuncture works on stimulating the nervous system to release endorphins to help deal with pain. It also uses neurotransmitters as "chemical messengers" between cells to allow the brain to send signals to the acupuncture point that has been needled.

Of course, you can still tell your partner that "they stuck pins in me", but understanding the relationship of acupuncture to what we may regard as "Western" medicine gives you a better understanding of just what is happening and why you are feeling better.

Acupuncture becoming more mainstream

As acupuncture became seen as a possible solution to a wide variety of issues – and believe me, some of the patients I have treated over the past nine years have presented with some extremely interesting issues! – it has become more popular as a treatment for dealing with all sorts of things.

But this book is about the *Guy Protocol* and how it works for menopausal symptoms. Of course I was going to name the protocol after me – and why not? After all, I wanted to make myself a little bit famous.[4]

---

4 Inspired by reading Penny Haslam's book, 'Make Yourself a Little Bit Famous.'

We have seen an increase in the popularity of acupuncture over the years as it has become more mainstream. It is also gaining momentum with additional clinical research coming out about its effectiveness. Partly this is down to an increased interest in acupuncture itself, but also due to a greater number of controlled studies giving meaningful data.

There is also another contributing factor in this equation — the rise of social media and the ability of people to connect with others around the globe who are searching for the same information or answers. This global connectivity means that the effectiveness of particular protocols can be shared across a wider demographic and the results reported on a far wider scale than was previously available.

On top of this, or perhaps in part because of this, there are many celebrities who now use acupuncture for a wide range of reasons. If social media is to be believed, it is rumoured that Sandra Bullock has acupuncture written into each of her acting contracts because she sees the benefits of regular acupuncture to balance her Qi and overall wellbeing whilst she is making movies. Back in 2007, Sheryl Crow stated in an interview with CNN that she had used acupuncture as part of her recovery from breast cancer.[5]

In addition, those of us in general practice are also seeing acupuncture being used more and more for mental health issues such as anxiety, stress and sadness. This coincides with, in Traditional Chinese Medicine terms, us becoming more and more "Yang" as a western society.

OK, so I did say I would keep this simple, so rather than try and explain the detail behind a society being more "Yang", let's just say that the traditional balance of yin and yang is currently disturbed in society, and the ensuing stresses and pressures are driving more and more people to re-examine

---

5 http://edition.cnn.com/2007/HEALTH/01/10/crow.cancer/index.html

their lifestyles and look for answers beyond the traditional Western medical practices of prescribing pills.

In summary, you can see that acupuncture, whilst having its roots firmly in Eastern culture, has crossed over into Western culture. The principles do make sense. There is nothing strange in there, no mumbo jumbo. Just some simple basics and an idea that helping keep the vital pathways around your body clear is good for you.

Millions of people around the world have acupuncture every day and wherever you look, you can find people who swear by it. And these days you don't have to look very hard. Even the NHS says acupuncture can be used in many NHS GP practices,[6] as well as in most pain clinics and hospices in the UK. Even my own GP did a foundation course in acupuncture after seeing the difference it made to my health.

I'm not getting as many hot flushes as I was before I started having acupuncture.

SH

Next time you are online, just try and Google "Does acupuncture work?" and see what comes top of the pile. Google is notorious for suppressing "quack" medical advice and even had an update to its algorithm in 2018 to help filter the results, so what you read at the top of the search results is now generally reliable medical information.

So, having established that acupuncture works and can work for a range of aliments, including hot flushes in menopausal women, the next big question is: "What is the *Guy Protocol*"?

---

6   https://www.nhs.uk/conditions/acupuncture/

CHAPTER FIVE

The Guy Protocol

Some things in life are just meant to be, some kind of happy accident perhaps. The story behind how I came to create the *Guy Protocol* probably sits in that category, as when I started life as an acupuncturist, I definitely didn't see this coming.

When I first qualified as an acupuncturist, I thought I would go down the cosmetic acupuncture route in the clinic. As part of the post graduate teaching I had been enthralled by it and after I'd seen the effects it could have on women I realised that this was exactly the kind of difference I wanted to make, helping women feel better about themselves without invasive procedures. I'd also seen the press reports about how some Hollywood A-listers were using it and in my mind, it was precisely the thing to bring to the well-heeled suburbs of leafy Cheshire.

Building pages on the website for cosmetic acupuncture was relatively straightforward, and as my husband had just started a company specialising in Search Engine Optimisation (SEO), getting them to rank highly on Google wasn't a problem. In no time, when you searched in Cheshire for Cosmetic Acupuncture, my website was top.

I also started to advertise locally for cosmetic acupuncture, using paid digital advertising, social media and some local publications, and I told all my patients about it. Cosmetic Acupuncture, to me at the time, was the thing that every woman needed. It was non-invasive, didn't rely on injections into your face and could show transformative differences almost immediately. I was fired up, ready to help educate the women of Cheshire, but there I was, ready for the wave of enquiries, and nothing happened.

In my head this was a bit of a blow. Lots of other acupuncture enquiries were coming in, but nothing for the type of acupuncture I really wanted to specialise in. I had thought that the rich and famous didn't need Botox, they needed acupuncture. However, I quickly realised that this simply wasn't the case, and on a day to day basis in the clinic I had to become more mainstream, treating patients for all kinds of aliments. Every day brought a new set of challenges and a different set of problems, but I slowly realised that most people, and particularly women, were coming to me for back issues, fertility issues, musculoskeletal difficulties and more straightforward (yet no less debilitating) troubles, like headaches. I found this to be hugely rewarding and I started to think about other things acupuncture could be used for to make a difference to people's lives.

It seemed like the universe was trying to tell me something.

About that same time as I was pondering the issue of not getting any enquiries for cosmetic acupuncture, one of my close friends, Shaun, was diagnosed with terminal cancer. This was a bitter blow to me as, working together for a number of years on a local Parish Council, we had become really close friends.

He wasn't the type of person to give up without a fight and he made sure his final years were filled with adventure and memories. Finally, however, when his body couldn't keep fighting any more, he ended up being cared for by the lovely people at St Luke's Hospice in Winsford, Cheshire. If you have a good memory, you will remember that it was Shaun who first suggested that I contact the hospice about acupuncture. He was receiving complementary therapies to try and help ease his suffering and the one thing he knew might help him and the one thing that was missing was acupuncture.

It's a funny old universe, isn't it, because if Shaun hadn't recommended that I contact the hospice, I don't think it was something I would ever have considered. Applying my training to a clinical situation like this, helping patients struggling with pain, either in a recovery plan after cancer treatments including surgery, or going through an end-of-life programme, had never crossed my mind. I'd been lucky and mostly spared this kind of situation in my life to this point, so to think I could apply acupuncture to this was something of a leap.

With Shaun's words ringing in my ears, I approached the team at St Luke's to see if they would consider adding acupuncture to the list of complementary therapies they provided for patients in the hospice. As luck would have it, they were not only interested but keen to add in someone with my skill set. So, late in 2012, I stepped through the doors of the hospice clinic to begin a new chapter in my acupuncture journey.

And what a journey it was! It soon became apparent that I was going to be treating a lot of people who were in a lot of pain. Some would never recover and were on end-of-life plans, and seeing them really affected me. What struck me however, was the stoicism of each and every one of them.

Knowing their bodies were being destroyed by cancer but still determined to fight to the last breath and grateful to anyone who would help them do so.

The main issues that people presented with at first were pain management and I spent some time perfecting a pain management protocol. But over the course of time, during the six years I spent working at the hospice, more and more patients were referred to me having been diagnosed with breast cancer.

Over 50 people a week die of breast cancer in the UK.

At first this was a trickle, but towards the end it was a constant stream, and I reckon that over the six years in St Luke's Hospice, up to 85% of my patients were referred to me after receiving treatment for breast cancer.

Breast cancer is a killer with 11,399 deaths attributable to the disease between 2015 and 2019,[7] making up 7% of total cancer deaths in the UK. That's over 2,800 deaths a year, or more tellingly, over 50 a week. And many of these patients, mostly women, end up having medical interventions in an effort to save their lives.

Typically, when faced with a breast cancer diagnosis, there are two main choices. Either have a mastectomy, after which is may be possible to have a reconstruction (although some women choose not to pursue this), or have a lumpectomy, where the affected tissue is surgically removed along with a large margin around it to ensure all the cancer is gone.

In both cases, this can then be followed with a course of chemotherapy and/or radiotherapy to sterilise the area around where the cancer was removed.

The end result, however, is that your body is deeply affected by whichever treatment you choose and the majority

---

7   https://www.cancerresearchuk.org/health-professional/cancer-statistics/statistics-by-cancer-type/breast-cancer/mortality

of patients find that there are the side effects of the drugs, the surgery or the subsequent treatments.

The good news is that with modern diagnostics and a countrywide screening programme, more women than ever are being diagnosed early and treated. As a consequence, survival rates are higher than they have even been. And outcomes can be improved even further if people seek medical help at the very first signs of breast cancer. Which gives me another opportunity to stand on my soapbox and shout:

Check your boobs, ladies AND gents – Regularly!

The women presenting for treatment at my clinic within the hospice had many similar symptoms, and in some respects, despite their differing stories and journeys, they all needed the same thing. Typically, women attending this clinic with me would present with hot flushes, night sweats, sleep disturbance, fatigue, foggy brain, aches and pains throughout the body, digestive issues and a range of other ailments.

> **"**
>
> *My sleep has much improved.*
> EC

Initially, I saw no similarities with this group of patients and menopause symptoms, and I would see them either individually or as part of a group acupuncture session. The sheer breadth of symptoms meant the connection wasn't immediately obvious. But as time went on, I realised that these women were experiencing similar symptoms, mostly as an aftereffect of breast surgery or a mastectomy. Almost everyone attending the clinic was presenting with the same hot flushes and the same night sweats, and almost all needed help with pain management after their breast surgery.

When it finally dawned on me that hot flushes were the most obvious presented symptom, I started to join the dots. Sleep disturbances, fatigue, mood swings and a foggy brain – this all sounded familiar, but where had I seen all these symptoms before?

Group therapy was an interesting area and one which, given the personal nature of the symptoms, I had assumed might not work so well. But I found groups beneficial, not only from a productivity point of view for me as the therapist, but it was also an overall therapeutic benefit to the patients. You know the old sayings "it's good to talk" or "a problem shared is a problem halved", well, right before my very eyes I could see bonds of friendships happening and patients getting so much more from their acupuncture sessions than just trying to help with their symptoms.

As I was now treating so many people on a weekly basis, I was able to build up a working knowledge of which acupuncture points worked best for certain situations. Over time I refined this to the point where I was able to measure positive outcomes from the clinical data of the majority of patients. Acupuncture was helping with breast cancer recovery symptoms such as hot flushes, sleep disturbances, mood swings and aches and pains, but it also became evident that these same issues were being suffered by patients going through the menopause. Finally, the penny had dropped.

As the *Menopausal Godmother*, I must have treated over a thousand women going through the menopause. Listening to the symptoms and what each patient is experiencing can sometimes be heartbreaking. In my field, we call this the "healing conversation" and just listening can make such a difference to someone. Those thousands of hours have given me a real insight into the menopause beyond my own personal experience. It has also provided me with the clarity to understand that whether naturally occurring or precipitated by some life change, the symptoms of breast cancer surgery recovery and menopause are remarkably similar.

The evolution of the Guy Protocol

Back in the clinic, with each new set of patients, I was able to experiment with different points and, whilst some were uniquely effective in some patients, the majority of people I treated responded well to the use of the same set of points on a consistent basis.

With this experimentation and refinement of acupuncture points, it wasn't too long before the *Guy Protocol* was born.

The Guy Protocol	
Tonify +	Reduce −
ST 36	SP6
KI3	SP9
	LIV2
Tonify − Clockwise to boost	
Reduce − Anticlockwise to reduce	

Now, you may not be familiar with some of the jargon here, but if you recall earlier in the book, I listed the different channels which we needle, such as spleen, liver and so on. In this illustration, you can see I needle Spleen 6 and 9 and Liver 2, Stomach 36 and Kidney 3. The "tonify" and "reduce" is turning the needle either clockwise or anti clockwise to crank up or lessen the effect of the needled point.

The points I chose were deliberately selected based on my experience of their effectiveness with other patients in other circumstances.

The first point I chose was Stomach 36 (St36), sometimes known as "leg 3 miles" for its reputed ability to enable ancient Chinese warriors to march an extra 3 miles after receiving treatment to this point. It's a really useful general acupuncture point, helping with energy, improving digestion, benefits the stomach and spleen and can help disperse stagnation in the body, such as constipation. It also helps with dizziness and fatigue and boosts the immune system and it was for these reasons, as well as its all-round abilities, that it was an obvious starting point.

The second point was Spleen 6 (Sp6) which is primarily used for gynaecological disorders and any issues with the uterus, so clearly this was a likely candidate. Typically, it helps to regulate hormones and as hot sweats are directly related to this, the point definitely needed to be included.

The next point was Spleen 9 (Sp9) which was chosen as it is a point that helps transport spleen Qi around the body so helps with abdominal pain, edema (swelling) and damp in the body. It's also helpful with knees and muscular issues in the lower limbs.

The fourth point was Kidney 3 (Ki3) which is mainly used to strengthen the lower back and is really good for night sweats and insomnia.

And finally, the fifth point was Liver 2 (Lv2) because this point is used to cool blood heat and therefore calms hot flushes. It also helps with anger, and as mood swings are often associated with menopause, this seemed to be a very useful point to try.

There is a real shortage of clinical data around acupuncture treatments generally, and especially around the issues of menopause, so it become important to find a way to not only test these treatments but to capture the data in a meaningful way. And so we conducted an independent assessment of the impact the *Guy Protocol* was having on my patients.

You can see in the data in the Appendix how the protocol helped women (and men) with hot flushes and pain relief. This study and research was taken over the period of a year and the evidence here is all independently verified and analysed.

66

My hot flushes are a lot less frequent and intense.
MB

I've decided to reproduce the *Guy Protocol* in this book exactly as it was published, as whilst it may appear clinical to some readers, it contains everything needed to demonstrate that this protocol works. My hope is that readers will be able to show this to their acupuncturist, who will easily be able to follow the points, and that other acupuncturists may use these to help alleviate the symptoms of hot flushes in their patients.

You can find the entire clinical evidence and protocol at the back of the book in the Appendix, but as parts of it may seem impenetrable, I'll summarise the key findings here.

The main issues presenting in the study

	(Number)
Hot flushes / sweats	*(41)*
Pain	*(17)*
Sleep problems	*(14)*
Other physical concerns / symptoms (e.g. headaches, arthritis)	*(9)*

- ■ **Hot flushes / sweats**
- ▨ **Pain**
- ▨ **Sleep problems**
- ■ **Other physical concerns / symptoms (e.g. headaches, arthritis)**

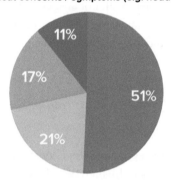

The predominant issue was hot flushes and sweats (51%), so naturally the protocol focused primarily on that area. The *Guy Protocol* has six points on both sides of the legs, and we treat bilaterally, meaning both sides of the body are used, with equal and opposite needles in each leg. The points were specifically chosen because they are all away from the upper body and this is important. It is essential not to needle around the area of surgery, especially if you are treating a lady after breast cancer.

Here is a real-life example of how I used the
Guy Protocol:

A 48-year-old lady had noticed a lump in her breast
whilst on holiday and was subsequently diagnosed with breast
cancer. She had two children at the time: one five-year-old
boy and one eleven-year-old girl. To that point, she had been
generally in good health and exercised regularly by teaching
karate to children. There was no family history of cancer.

This story is not unusual and most women find their life
turned upside down by this type of discovery and diagnosis.

Following diagnosis and consideration of all the
different options available, she opted for a lumpectomy and
had surgery to remove the lump in her breast. After that she
underwent chemotherapy and was subsequently prescribed
Tamoxifen.

Tamoxifen is the standard treatment in premenopausal
women with hormone positive breast cancer and is also
routinely used in women who have been through the
menopause. Tamoxifen is usually given after surgery for
up to ten years to prevent the recurrence of cancer,
although some women take it for two to three years before
switching to a different type of medication knows as an
"aromatase inhibitor".

Tamoxifen is used to block oestrogen from reaching the
cancer cells, meaning the cancer either grows very slowly
or stops growing altogether. The side effects of this drug,
however, can mimic menopause, causing hot flushes and
night sweats, depression, palpations and mood swings, and
mental restlessness.

Earlier research into the use of acupuncture in this type
of situation had proved that this type of intervention could
create a natural response in the body to produce an anti-
cancer immune response.

So, when she presented in the hospice, I gave her six treatments, during which in each session she was treated using the *Guy Protocol*.

The protocol was based around the common symptoms presenting in most breast cancer patients and designed to alleviate the symptoms of hot flushes.

Needling was done bilaterally on both legs and as I said earlier, I avoided the upper body as sometimes there is the chance of lymphedema. Lymphedema is a swelling of the lymph nodes in the armpit that sometimes happens after surgery or radiotherapy. Lymphedema framework guidelines recommend avoiding puncturing the skin to reduce the risk of infection.

In my initial diagnosis I had noted that the patient's tongue was dry and cracked. From a Chinese Medical standpoint, that means that the body was "thirsty". Her pulses were weak and given that she was on Tamoxifen, this wasn't a surprise.

According to Chinese medicine, Tamoxifen tends to deplete the kidney yin (the cooling function) and so acupuncture attempts to restore the yin, thereby controlling the hot flushes. Chinese medicine generally maintains that acupuncture is not strong enough to get rid of the cancer by itself, but it is effective in promoting the flow of Qi and aims to help the body recover and to minimise the chance of recurrence. It was with this in mind that I began my treatments.

It's useful to show you here exactly what I did for her over the course of six weeks and the observations of her response to the treatment.

What is particularly interesting is the notes below the needling points. These were made at the time I gave the treatments and show you a clear progression over a six-week period, from the woman struggling with hot flushes and night sweats to being completely free of them and being able to enjoy a full night's sleep once again.

Guy Protocol treatment and observations

Treatment	Timing	Points and Observations
1		**Guy Protocol** **Spleen 6, 9 liv2, reduced, st36, ki3 tonified** Although a little needle phobic, once a few needles were placed she was more relaxed. Needles stayed in for twenty-five minutes.
2	7 days later	**Spleen 6, 9 liv2, reduced, st36, ki3 tonified** Patient still experiencing hot flushes, no particular change/still sleep disturbances. Needles stayed in for twenty-five minutes.
3	7 days later	**Spleen 6, 9 liv2, reduced, st36, ki3 tonified** Patient experiencing hot flushes but comments they are about 20-30% less frequent and not as severe. Sleeping much better. Needles stayed in for twenty-five minutes.
4	7 days later	**Spleen 6, 9 liv2, reduced, st36, ki3 tonified** Patient experiencing hot flushes but comments they are about 50-60% less frequent and not as severe. Sleeping much better. Needles stayed in for twenty-five minutes.
5	7 days later	**Spleen 6, 9 liv2, reduced, st36, ki3 tonified** No flushes other than feeling a little warm, sleeping well. Needles stayed in for twenty-five minutes.
6	7 days later	**Spleen 6, 9 liv2, reduced, st36, ki3 tonified** No flushes. Needles stayed in for twenty-five minutes.

The end result was a wonderful outcome for her in that she experienced a reduction in the number and duration of the hot flushes every week during the first three weeks of treatment and, after her fourth treatment, the hot flushes stopped completely.

Of course, this is not the end of the story, but it is the beginning of the end. This patient, like so many others I see, simply needs to have intermittent "top up" treatments of acupuncture to keep the Qi in balance to ensure that the hot sweats are not the debilitating nuisance they were before.

And this example is not unusual. I have used these points on hundreds of women and experienced the same results – the end of the misery of hot flushes and night sweats.

This is backed up by the results of the independent clinical study. Once the study had finished, the data was analysed and some excellent outcomes were reported. Here are the responses the participants gave to the question "What were the most important aspects for you [of the Acupuncture Clinic set up for the Guy Protocol]?"

Improvements noted after treatment in the study

	(Number)
Improvement in hot flushes / sweats	(17)
Acupuncturist	(13)
Being able to relax / feel at ease	(12)
Company / group / making new friends	(11)
Increased confidence / well-being / feeling more positive	(10)
Improved sleep	(8)
Talking / chatting / being listened to	(7)

As you can see, the study showed that acupuncture and the *Guy Protocol* made a real difference to the lives of those participating in the study. Because of the similarity of the symptoms of people being treated for breast cancer and those going through menopause, it was obvious to me that the *Guy Protocol* could help some of the millions of women going through the menopause each year.

But that's not everything. If only it were that simple, then there would be a lot more acupuncturists in the country! As the *Menopausal Godmother*, I have seen the positive effects that making small changes in lifestyle, diet and exercise can have on women and the impact these changes have. So, after we've heard about exercise and nutrition next, I'll pick up on what you can also be doing to help yourself through menopause.

Menopause, Fitness and Nutrition

When you turn the page to the nutrition and fitness chapter, it is so easy to think "not another diet plan with the miracle solutions!" I would have been inclined to agree, until I met Emma Wilson of *Emma Wilson Fitness*, the co-author of this chapter along with Mindy Cowap! Emma has created a programme (*My Time for Change by Emma Wilson Fitness*) that is a holistic approach to your health and wellbeing, where food and fitness are at the bottom of the priority list in your search for that zest for life that often is cloaked by changes to your emotional, mental and physical self as you enter the perimenopausal and menopausal years.

> *Simply changing my diet has given me more energy and makes it easier to deal with the way the menopause makes me feel.*
>
> EG

I'm delighted that I managed to convince Mindy Cowap and Emma Wilson to contribute this next chapter to the book.

Not only do they think along the same lines as me when it comes to these matters, but they are both focused on helping menopausal women make the most of their menopause. Here's what they have to say.

Mindy's story

I joined the *My Time for Change* programme in September 2018, having fought with emotional and weight issues for most of my adult life, then entering the perimenopause stage. The programme changed my life! Within 12 months, at 46, I had lost more than 5 stone, trekked the Sahara Desert (raising £11,000 for St Luke's Hospice), climbed Snowdon, learnt to ski and to wakeboard and discovered (not even re-discovered) a *zest for life* that I didn't even know I should have had! As I ran up 364 steep-steps daily on our family holiday to Mallorca, I knew I'd hit a pinnacle of happiness when my 9-year-old son said to me, "Mummy I want to be as fit and healthy as you." Within that year, I had morphed from a middle-aged-morbidly-obese-exercise-phobe into an inspiration to my children!

Emma educated me on how to fuel my body with real food, so I no longer felt like I was on a "diet" and therefore missing out! She taught me how to move efficiently so that I didn't need to feel punished by exercise over long periods of time. And she demonstrated that the hormonal changes, the emotional overwhelm and anxiousness, could be managed by the food I ate, the types of exercise I did and how much water I drank! Learning all of this whilst part of a community of women who were also seeking the answers to changes in their lives was totally inspiring and lifestyle changing.

I hadn't realised that much of what was happening to me was menopause related, in fact I hadn't ever talked about the menopause before! I had assumed that it would be my fifties before I needed to even consider this. I had always been overweight, so noticing physical changes was part and parcel of my ever-yoyoing weight problem, the loss of mental clarity at times was making me anxious, assuming I was regressing to a point of no-return and the irrational reactions at times I put down to other stresses in my life. Emma has since taught me that these feelings are potentially only 3 of around 34 menopausal symptoms that I could demonstrate! That in fact a holistic approach to food, fitness, stress, sleep and much more can help you cope and manage any of these 34 symptoms, if not overcome them.

I am such an advocate of the programme, of the happiness, health and the air it has breathed into my life, that I approached Emma to ask if I could become her business partner. I wanted to help her shout about the programme from the roof tops, to help women recognise that they are not alone in how they are feeling, that they don't have to accept their size, shape, aches, pains and that they too can be educated about helping themselves to reach optimum wellbeing and restore hormonal balance by making subtle changes to lifestyle. Fortunately for me, Emma said yes, so since early 2020, *My Time for Change* became a duo!

Mindy ☺

Where it all began

Hi, I'm Emma Wilson creator of *My Time for Change* and *Emma Wilson Fitness*.

I am a UK-based fitness and health coach with a natural passion for helping people feel the very best they can.

I've always enjoyed sport and keeping fit, but after a

prolapsed disk injury in 1999, I had 5 years of pain and generally feeling robbed of my functioning body. The lack of activity, coupled with a stressful and sedentary job, led to considerable weight gain and some emotional challenges.

So, after the birth of my daughter in 2005 (when I was age 32) I decided to take things into my own hands and get myself stronger and fitter. That path brought me to the realisation that there was something missing for people who were starting out exercising or had exercised previously and been injured. A place and person that made them feel included, accomplished and a success when it comes to activity.

With that in mind, I embarked on a career change, went back to education and in 2006 *Emma Wilson Fitness* was born! In the early days, my focus was ante and postnatal exercise prescription with focus on helping new mums get back into shape. Little did I realise at the time, that this knowledge and expertise overlaps so much with the menopausal body too.

Since those early days, my portfolio has continued to expand, offering a wide and varied fitness programme, along with personal training for all ages and abilities. From those that need a little TLC to those that want a beasting!

In 2014 (age 41), I started to notice changes in my own body that intrigued me. Feeling thicker around the middle, not getting the same results from my workouts, mood change and sleep patterns. I started to delve deeper into women's health, hormones and nutrition. *My Time for Change* was created in 2017, an online wellbeing and weight-loss programme for women 35 and over. My ultimate goal and wish is that every woman can feel as happy and healthy as they can be. The programme gives women the knowledge so that they can make informed decisions to shift that stubborn unwanted mid-riff and improve their mental and emotional wellbeing. Perimenopause can be tough at times, but when you know how to handle it, you can be energised, resilient and feel your best self.

The vast majority of who I talk to and see are female, but my classes and the principles behind both my fitness arm and health hub apply to everyone the world over.

I think that life is about balance, not denying yourself what you enjoy, having a little of what you fancy and I fully believe that age is just a number.

I love helping people achieve their goals, whatever they may be.

Within a few years I was fortunate enough to find the strength within me to make change. Changes that would affect family life in order to protect my mental health, but also changes that would impact on my physical shape and overall wellbeing. I took a holistic approach and sought a number of alternative therapies to help build my resolve to become the woman I am!

At 47 (2020), I feel I am at the peak of health, but every day is a new opportunity to make improvements, however small they may be. I have found true happiness from within and am rewarded daily and thrive on helping women to live the lives they love! My online programme has now changed hundreds of women's lives. I never tire of the positive impacts that making small lifestyle changes can have on someone's life!

Emma x

So why could it be YOUR time for change?

At a time when our hormones are starting to alter and changes physically, mentally and emotionally begin to happen, it is important to understand why what we put into our bodies and how we move can affect our hormones, our sleep, memory, emotions and so much more, particularly as women from the age of 35 upwards. These hormone changes can really impact on our wellbeing and zest for life.

The programme is about making small lifestyle tweaks. Being given the tools to understand fact from fiction about what's really health giving and healthful, being guided so you can dispel diet myths that have perhaps kept you chained to foods rather than feeling liberated, being supported so you can feel confident to move in a new and effective way to affect your metabolism and ever changing body, getting results you truly deserve by working smarter and not harder so you don't feel hindered in your quest for good health and a better body shape. All this contributes and affects your sleep, hormone balance and health markers in a hugely positive way. Health markers such as type 2 diabetes, obesity or high blood pressure can be managed or reversed. Understanding how to make these changes without feeling like you are deprived by a "diet" or enslaved to fitness is how *My Time for Change* is unique.

The vital link between immunity, digestive function and gut health – are you looking after your second brain?

We all know that looking after our health and wellbeing should be at the top of our agenda. However, what is often overlooked, when it comes to our health, is our digestive system.

The digestive tract is critical to your health because 70-80% of your entire immune system is located in your digestive tract.

Your digestive tract is lined with good bacteria called probiotics which support your body's ability to absorb nutrients and fight infection. The good bacteria that live in our intestines help prime our gut immune tissue to recognise whether new invaders are friend or foe.

In addition to the impact on our immune system, our digestive system is the second largest part of our central nervous system. It is located in our gut and therefore the gut is fondly known as our second brain. Our gut is also responsible for creating around 90% of our serotonin levels (one of the happy hormones) and therefore may have significant impact on our brain function and mood.

There are many health issues that can be connected with gut function and gut health, such as thyroid imbalance, chronic fatigue, joint pain, skin complaints, and inflammatory illness such as arthritis. Inflammation in the gut can lead to auto-immune illness like type 2 diabetes, obesity, heart disease, colitis, Crohn's disease, eczema, anxiety, depression, IBS, allergies... to name a few.

The secret to good gut health is all about balancing out the good and bad bacteria (known as microbiome) in your digestive system. Bacteria is a living, breathing thing; we have to show it premium care.

Numerous factors have a positive impact on gut health, including a nutritious, varied diet and regular exercise to stimulate digestion. Getting sufficient sleep is particularly important as this is when our body does its repairing, but it's also when our immune cells return to our lymph nodes. When a lymph node is presented with a "new" foreign body from other immune cells it learns to recognise them and attack.

The good and friendly bacteria are commonly called probiotics. Consuming rich probiotic foods or taking a good probiotic supplement will help keep those good bacteria topped up as it's a real balancing act keeping those good bacteria in plentiful supply.

What about prebiotics? Well these are non-digestible fibres that probiotics need to feed on, you may also know this as inulin. If you haven't got the right food for your good bacteria, those probiotics are unlikely to be able to do their job. So consuming rich prebiotic food or a good prebiotic supplement will help.

Various environmental and dietary habits can affect the quality of our gut bacteria, so it's important not to treat pre and probiotics as a "magic pill" and cure-all. We have to be responsible and so we limit our probiotic killers.

What are the top killers of probiotics (our gut's good bacteria)?

- Overuse of prescription antibiotics
- Sugar
- Genetically modified (GMO) foods
- Emotional Stress
- Medications
- Alcohol
- Lack of exercise
- Smoking
- Poor sleep habits

EASY EVERYDAY TIPS

Drink a minimum of 2 litres of water a day.

Include protein in every meal.

Aim for 7-9 vegetables every day,
minimum of 2 which are dark,
green and leafy.

Super easy and healthy recipe

Chicken Skewers & Tumble (serves 4)

(Can substitute chicken with fish or vegetable skewers)

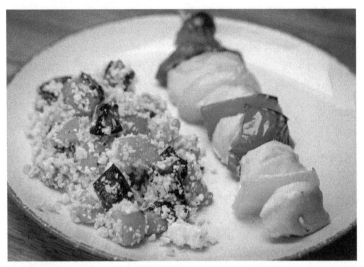

Ingredients

- 500g diced chicken
- 1 green, 1 yellow and 1 red pepper cut into chunks
- 150g peeled & diced sweet potato
- 125g peeled and diced butternut squash
- 3 tablespoons coconut oil, melted
- 2 tablespoons butter, melted
- Salt and pepper
- 2 tbsp pumpkin seeds
- 1 head cauliflower blitzed to rice in a food processor
- Drizzle of olive oil
- 100g feta

Method

1. Preheat the oven to 200˚c
2. Place the sweet potato and butternut squash on a roasting tray and drizzle with the coconut oil and melted butter. Season with salt and pepper.
3. Roast for 35 minutes until soft.
4. Place the diced chicken and peppers onto 4 skewers. Alternate 1 piece of pepper and 1 piece of chicken along the skewer.
5. Place the chicken skewers on a separate roasting tray, drizzle with olive oil and cook in the oven for 30 minutes – or cook on the BBQ!
6. Chop the feta into small pieces.
7. Pour the pumpkin seeds into the oven tray with the sweet potato and butternut squash and place back in the oven for 2 minutes.
8. Then add the cauliflower rice to the sweet potato, butternut squash and pumpkin seeds, stir to create the tumble and place back in the oven for 5 minutes.
9. Remove all from the oven, drizzle the tumble with olive oil and stir in the feta.
10. Serve immediately. Also delicious chilled.

Exercise – Mid-section movement for mid-life

All weights are optional

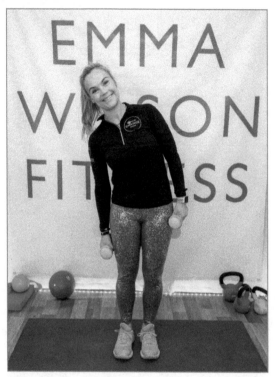

Exercise 1:

1. Stand up tall, feet natural hip-width apart.
2. Hold weight in each hand (this can be bottles, tins or bags of shopping).
3. Keeping belly button pulled back to spine, keeping shoulders square (imagine being sandwiched between 2 panes of glass), slide one hand down the right thigh, keeping arms straight, and then back to centre.
4. Repeat 10 times on the right side, repeat 10 times on the left side.

Exercise 2:

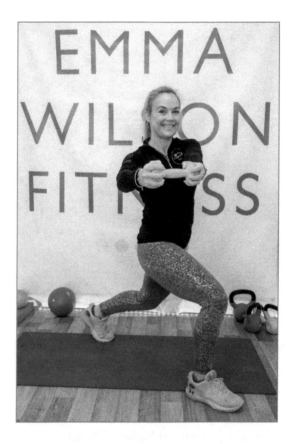

1. Stand up tall, feet natural hip-width apart.
2. Holding a weight at your chest, lunge forward with right leg, extend arms straight out in front and rotate both arms, keeping straight, around to the right. Bring back to centre, step back the right leg, bring the weight back to your chest. Repeat 10 times.
3. Repeat on left leg.

Exercise 3:

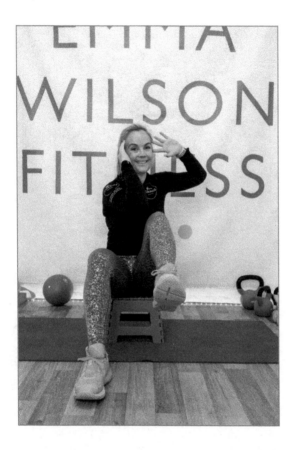

1. Using a chair, sit tall on the edge of the seat pad, ensuring that hips, knees and ankles are at right angles with each other. Sit up tall.
2. Bring fingertips to temples and open up the elbows. Take a breath in through the nose, and as you breathe out through the mouth rotate opposite elbow to opposite inside knee. Alternate each side 20 times.

Exercise 4:

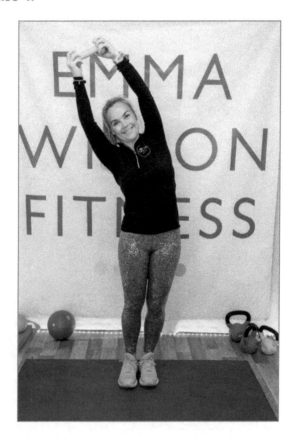

1. Standing tall, feet together.
2. Take both arms straight above your head, holding a weight (optional) drop shoulders away from ears. In metronome fashion tick tock from left to right, bending at the waist, always keeping the hands shoulder-width apart. (Think muffin top). Tick tock for 1 minute.

Exercise 5:

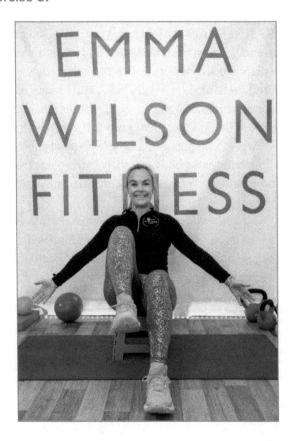

1. Using a chair, sit tall on the edge of the seat pad, ensuring that hips, knees and ankles are at right angles with each other. Sit up tall.
2. Drive knees and thighs directly up towards the chest, high knee marching, breathing out through the mouth as the knees drive up. Repeat for 1 minute.

A magical pill?

The *My Time for Change* journey is not a magical pill, you still have to be consistent, persistent and accountable. However, when you are equipped with the knowledge, supported and motivated on a daily basis, and embraced and inspired by a community of like-minded women, the monthly programme feels like as close as you can get! You live the life you love, whilst understanding how if you fuel effectively and move efficiently, your body can thrive, overcome health markers and whatever your age, be the woman you arrived on this planet to be!

Thank you to the *Menopausal Godmother*, Emma Guy, for including us in your book. We have a common goal to show that the menopausal years can be embraced and thrived within! Stronger together!

Emma and Mindy xx

www.emmawilsonfitness.co.uk
www.mytimeforchange.co.uk

CHAPTER SEVEN

Hints and Tips From Other Godmothers

I n modern day society, we are bombarded with lots of diet and lifestyle choices, whether it's via social media, in the local supermarket or at the gym. We seem to be taking our health and wellbeing more seriously. We even have so called "influencers" who thousands if not millions follow on social media channels.

In my search to help you deal with your menopause, I would like to introduce you to experts in a range of specialisms, each who has some top tips for you.

Oh, and if you want to hear a bit more from them (which I am sure you will after hearing what they have to say), their contact details are at the back of the book.

Let's hear from some of our other Godmothers.

Reflexology – Sharron Roughton

Reflexology is a complementary therapy aimed at supporting the whole person, accessing the body systems via the feet or hands. The body is mapped on to the whole foot, and each area represents a corresponding area of the body. For example, the area corresponding to the brain is located on the underside and tip of the toes. Reflexology connects with various reflex points on the feet, and these pathways are connected via the central nervous system and the brain.

As a therapist, we are taught to connect with the whole person and incorporate physical and mental health and wellbeing throughout a treatment session, using our thoughts of intention for healing and an energetic connection.

Our bodies are a complicated network of chemicals and electrical messages constantly receiving and sending coded instructions via the central nervous system. These chemical messages are instructions from the brain and the endocrine system to release hormones throughout the body. When we are starting out in life and when we approach our teenage years these hormones begin to work overtime and increase their levels, preparing our bodies for adulthood.

As we age, this changes again as we come to the later years of our reproductive life. I refer to this time as Menopause Transition, and it has been described as perimenopause. Often women do not realise they have entered this phase; it can be subtle and women may not notice any significant changes.

One of the main symptoms of perimenopause and menopause is anxiety. In my experience, almost all women suffer from anxiety. It is a symptom that is often overlooked, and not talked about enough. Menopause for many women can be a very difficult time, and my own experience was one of lack of understanding and worry as I did not feel myself.

I decided to specialise in women's health and this aspect in particular as I have seen so many women affected by anxiety. Reflexology is an effective way to manage and improve these symptoms. It resets the body and brings balance to irregular body messages, and many clients have reported their outlook and self-worth improves considerably after just a 1-2 sessions.

Reflexology is used and adapted to every person's needs for each treatment, and is very effective in regulating body systems — this includes: improving sleep; reducing anxiety and low mood; regulating hormones; and reducing the symptoms many women experience during this life transition.

My top tips for anyone transitioning through menopause would be to try to keep the bedroom cool, wear loose layers and drink plenty of water. Listen to your body and, if you need to rest, then do so. Keep a diary if it helps to keep track of your symptoms and seek help. Talk about your feelings with your partner, friend or GP. You are not alone.

There is a great deal you can do to help yourself, one of which is reflexology. Clients have reported a more regulated cycle, fewer mood swings, reduced hot flashes, improved sleep patterns, less anxiety and improved wellbeing. Many women continue to feel the benefits of reflexology sessions by maintaining regular treatments. It is a natural, safe, relaxing and effective treatment, suitable for all.

Massage and Aromatherapy – Steph Fox

Aromatherapy is a holistic treatment using essential oils to promote balance and harmony with mind and body. There are many benefits and it has become one of the most requested treatments in beauty.

As the word suggests, aromatherapy means:
Aroma – a pleasant sweet smell of fragrance.
Therapy – healing treatment serving to improve or maintain health.

The use of essential oils and massage helps to maintain optimum health, especially in menopause. Menopause is a time of transition that involves changes in hormone levels. You can experience symptoms such as: anxiety, sleepless nights, restlessness, mood swings and hot flushes. Aromatherapy massage accompanied with the power of essential oils and plant extracts can help ease these symptoms.

Here are a few of my favourites:
- Clary sage – acts as an antidepressant.
- Bergamot – is a natural mood booster; it promotes feelings of energy and cheerfulness.
- Geranium – is a natural uplifter and relieves depression.
- Lavender – reduces stress, depression, anxiety and improves your sleep.

When blending your own oil at home you must make sure you use a carrier oil first then a few drops of chosen essential oil. Even better, why not book yourself a massage with your local beautician.[8]

Hypnotherapy – Rosemary Heaton

Gone are the days when people thought that going under hypnosis may lead to a loss of control, that the individual could be made to mimic a chicken or eat an onion raw at the hypnotist's command. In fact, it is quite the opposite.

Hypnotherapy has helped many women empower themselves during menopause, to achieve some control over symptoms that are often debilitating, particularly those dreaded hot sweats!

---

8   Please note that if you are using aromatherapy oils you must ensure that you carefully follow the instructions supplied with them. If you are unsure, then seek professional advice before using them.

A study carried out by Etkins et al (2013)[9] over 12 weeks compared a group of menopausal women undertaking hypnotherapy to a group that did not. Results demonstrated that the hypnotherapy group had 74% fewer hot flushes, compared with 17% fewer amongst the other women. Evidence from this study showed that the hypnosis group reported less disturbed or unrestful sleep.

It should be noted that hypnosis is not a replacement for hormone therapy, which is said to be more effective. However, hypnotherapy is a successful and well-evidenced alternative for those looking for a natural way to help at such a difficult time, which will also promote relaxation, peaceful sleep, and motivation.

Top Tip:

In my experience, a lot of women suffer with a low confidence as a result of menopause. That could be related to weight gain etc. It's therefore really important to have ACCEPTANCE of yourself and who you've become. Acknowledge your life experiences, challenges, and achievements. This helps you move forward in a positive way.

Style coach – Yifan Nairn

Going through the menopause does NOT mean you're past your prime or old. On the contrary, it's the perfect time to re-evaluate your priorities and find your true style. When you look good, you feel good. When you feel good about yourself, your confidence will shine through, no matter what age you are!

Your body is going through another change, just like it did through adolescence or childbirth. Embrace the change,

9 https://www.ncbi.nlm.nih.gov/pmc/articles/PMC3556367/

get to know your body shape and learn how to dress it so you feel most comfortable and confident.

Choosing the right fabrics, such as cotton, bamboo, or fast drying fabrics, can help you feel cool when hot flushes strike. Master layering skills so you can easily remove some layers if your body temperature increases.

Colours are mood enhancers and can put a spring in your step instantly. Instead of "hiding", wear what makes your eyes sparkle and skin radiant — although you might want to pay attention to whether your clothes show sweat patches easily if you get hot flushes!

Above all, experiment with styles that you couldn't wear before and have fun!

Reset framework – Naomi Gilmour

Life can certainly through us curve balls! I can talk firsthand (and often do) about life challenges, having experienced quite a few! I know like most, I want to embrace life, I want to laugh more and I honestly believe that happiness does lie within us and that when we start to search outside of ourselves to find our happy it doesn't come, because we truly have to find that within.

That's why I want to share with you a really simple mindset reframing tool to help you cope with life curve balls and build your inner happy.

I want you to think about those really tough times we have in life, where we feel sad and we can feel lost and overwhelmed, or where we are stressed out. We can feel like we want to just stay in bed and put the duvet back over our heads. Everything can feel overwhelming and just too hard.

But on the flip side, we can have joyous times too! We can be hanging out with friends, feeling healthy, having fun, feeling loved, and having togetherness in our lives, experiencing inner peace, calm, and feeling a sense of inner happy.

But in-between these two states there is a whole spectrum of feelings that we can work through in life.

So let's talk affirmations. Affirmations are a super powerful tool that you can use in your everyday life. Because what we tell ourselves is really what we become.

If you get up in the morning and look in the mirror and you say, "I feel fat. I feel ugly. I feel tired. My skin is ageing," you're going to reinforce all the negative stuff and make yourself feel that way; you're going to feel crap. So let's flip that around.

One of the first things that I do to shift my mood is to use sticky notes! Actually putting different affirmations around my home. Telling myself I feel beautiful, or simply, today I am enough.

"I am enough" is a big one. We are all enough.

We are all beautifully, imperfectly perfect.

I'm going to share this fabulous excerpt from *The One Minute Millionaire* by Victor Hansen:

"Today I am enough.

I am smart enough.

Wise enough.

Clever enough.

Resourceful enough.

Able enough.

Confident enough.

I am connected to enough people to accomplish my heart's desire.

I have enough ideas to pull off magic and miracles.

Enough is all I need.

Enough is all I have.

I have more than enough.

As I do all that I can do I'm able to do more and more and I'm excited to be alive.

I rejoice and re-choice every day to make my life better.

I'm happy, healthy, prosperous, successful, rich, loving, loved, beloved.

I'm comfortable with myself, so I am comfortable with others.

I confidently greet each day with a smile on my face and love in my heart and everyone who meets me is warmed by the radiance of my attitude.

I work on my attitude continuously.

I read positive, inspiring, uplifting books.

I listen to audio tapes and CDs during my driving and exercise times.

I associate with friendly, caring, nurturing people who are involved, doing important things, and the people whom I associate want more for me than I want for myself.

The projects which I'm involved wow my soul.

I am passionately on purpose to do good, be good and help others do the same.

I am enough. I have enough. I do enough."

You are all enough. Everybody is enough.

Alongside "enoughness" there are an abundance of affirmations you can search up online. Pop them on a sticky note on your mirror, or order yourself some cards — there's everything from animal guidance, positive power thought cards to funny light hearted messages to choose from. I have quite a collection on my desk and use them daily. Take a minute for yourself, breathe, choose yourself a card, read it, and repeat it! Revisit it throughout rest of your day, and every day, whatever it takes! The more you read it the more you will believe and mindset is crucial to wellbeing, feeling good and believing in yourself to create your inner happy!

Menopause and Mindfulness – Toni Mackenzie

Most women become programmed to feel negative about menopause, expecting it to be difficult and focusing upon it being "the end" rather than embracing it as a transformation towards a positive new beginning. When you're thinking negatively you create feelings of low mood, anxiety and stress, which create and increase physical symptoms. Changing your mindset and adopting a positive attitude can not only release those negative feelings, it can also release or relieve any associated physical symptoms.

If you keep telling yourself that something's going to be difficult, physically or emotionally, then that's likely to be your experience. To become aware of your thoughts, place a rubber band around your wrist and every time you see it throughout the day, pause and notice what you're thinking. If it's negative, ping the rubber band, command your mind to stop the thought and change it for a positive one that makes you feel good. Within days of consistently doing this your mind will learn that it's no longer controlling you and you have taken back control of it.

More often than not, most people are dwelling on the past, often creating feelings of regret, resentment or guilt, or thinking about what might go wrong in the future, creating anxiety, worries and fears. Mindfulness involves bringing yourself into the present moment, stopping that train of thought and being fully present.

When you're aware only of the present moment, your mind and body can become still and you can feel peace and ease. You can practice it anytime, anywhere – when you're out walking, focus on your immediate surroundings and feel your feet on the floor; in the shower – feel the warm water, smell the fragrance, enjoy the experience, rather than being in your head. Post sticky notes in the car, on mirrors, doors – anywhere you'll see them and remember to pause and be present throughout the day.

Menopause and Medicine – Dr Gill Barham

As a former nurse and now holistic health practitioner, I have had a long and quite extreme experience with the menopause. I noticed changes at 39, but things really kicked off big time after a hysterectomy as 45. Throughout, I have been devoted to finding and recommending natural ways to combat the sometimes debilitating symptoms I and many other women encounter. I did use HRT for a while but was put off by the scare stories. Of the 40 symptoms I have listed on my website, I think I am personally familiar with all but about 5!

There is much that can be done to alleviate some, if not all, if we look from the viewpoint of building health rather than treating the menopause as a disease. As with most other physical or emotional changes, in my experience, taking a holistic approach by trying out treatments, supplements and therapies that suit you personally is the key to success and some of them are highlighted in this chapter.

However, to achieve a sense of true wellbeing, all this has to be underpinned by good nutrition and building a healthy gut. So most of my work with menopausal women starts with re-establishing a good clean eating programme and a balanced microbiome. Most of it is common sense, but I am blessed to be "in" on the latest clinically trialled programmes and quality products that transform the lives of women who are open to lifestyle changes and want to make the most of their "wisdom" years.

Here are my 10 top tips in terms of natural supplementation and food:

1. Take an omega 3 supplement to help with the production of oestrogen and for heart, bone and brain health.
2. Eat foods made from individual ingredients – in other words, no processed foods, instead cooking from scratch.
3. Try to source local, in season and organic produce.
4. Buy only high quality supplements and take advice from a nutritional therapist or naturopath so you don't waste your money.
5. Take a magnesium supplement or bathe in Epsom salts for menopause health.
6. Drink lots of spring or filtered water every day – aim for 2 litres.
7. Totally cut out the known triggers – caffeine, alcohol, dairy, sugar and wheat – for at least a month to alleviate symptoms and only reintroduce one at a time so you can monitor effects.
8. Try herbal or targeted nutraceuticals (ask me for details).
9. Build your immune system with daily Vitamin D3, Zinc.
10. Consider doing my 21-day microbiome reset programme
    All this definitely makes a huge difference.

However, here's the thing. I am now 59, and up until 6 months ago, my symptoms were still getting in the way of me being able to live the life I want. What changed?

I developed vaginal atrophy. This is the thinning and shortening of all the organs and tissues around that area. This can result in discomfort, itching, pain, urinary problems, painful or impossible sex, loss of libido (no surprise there), bleeding and other vulval conditions.

Sadly, no amount of good nutrition or supplementation was going to help this and so I started to look at topical HRT. I learned that new transdermal (through the skin) versions are not only safe but protect us as we age from osteoporosis, heart disease, diabetes and dementia, with evidence that even women with family histories of breast or ovarian cancer can be prescribed in appropriate amounts by an experienced menopause specialist. I now use two forms and my life has been transformed.

Gill supports and guides women towards embracing their midlife by sharing her own and others stories and expertise on her podcast Radiant Menopause.

Skincare in the Menopause – Gerard and Joanna Lambe

None of us want to get any older but it's better than the alternative!

Menopause and perimenopause (typically 3-4 years before periods stop) is a time when hormone levels change significantly, especially oestrogen. Low oestrogen levels lead to dry skin due to reduced oil production as well as decreased collagen turnover that can lead to drooping and sagging. At this time, it can seem that your jowls and crow's feet arrive overnight!

So what can you do? Well first, make sure any products you are using are not drying out your skin – creamy cleansers are now better for you than foam or gels that would remove precious moisture. Now more than ever, your moisturising routine is key to your skincare regime, so consider changing to a heavier and more hydrating formula. Added to this, a cream or foundation containing a SPF should be a daily routine (even on overcast days) as sun damage can lead to age spots and more wrinkles. Aim for SPF 30 and use it daily.

Anything else that can help? Thankfully, yes. Retinoids are a family of products which have been used for many years to improve skin quality. They help to repair skin and improve collagen production and your blood supply, but some formulations can be drying, so read reviews and pick a product that works for your skin.

Don't forget to look after the back of your hands too, especially if you enjoy the outdoors, and again use a moisturiser containing SPF on them, plus wear gloves when you can.

General overall wellbeing is important to attend to as well, and a heathy diet and exercise plan will boost your blood supply, lower stress levels and improve your immune system. If exercise were a pill, we would all take one every day!

Finally, remember to enjoy this phase of your life too as every day counts.

Hair and the Menopause – Paula and Nicola

Many women notice changes to their bodies during menopause, and the skin and hair are key areas where these changes are most noticeable.

Your skin can become dehydrated and appear more wrinkled, and your hair can suffer dreadfully. As hairdressers, we notice these changes, sometimes even before the customer does. From our experience, here are a few top tips to help keep your hair in excellent condition:

- Drink lots of water to help keep the scalp and hair hydrated.
- Shampoo less often to help the hair from drying out (let the natural oils do their thing).

- Deep conditioners are great for putting moisture back into hair.
- HRT is great to help reduce hair loss. This is caused by the lowered levels of hormones and HRT replaces them.
- Protein makes your hair grow quicker; check your diet contains plenty of protein.
- Sage tablets have been shown to help reduce hot sweats.
- Try as best you can to keep cool, because sweat makes your hair dry and also causes your colour to fade quicker.
- Lost hair WILL grow back after the menopause but may not be as thick as it once was.
- Because of the hormone change, you may start to develop reactions or allergies to hair colour products. So, a skin test is recommended if you start to show any signs of a reaction. The darker the colour, the more likely the reactions because the colour that is put into your hair molecules fills the cortex of the hair shaft, unlike lighter colours where they are taken out.

And that's it! Remember, you can still look fabulous through menopause; just talk with your hairdresser about colours, products and styles as well as how to look after your hair during this time.

Make up in menopause – Charlotte Carney

I've been a professional makeup artist for around 3 years, although I've always loved makeup long before I considered it a job! My specialty is bridal and natural glam. I love to make women look beautiful and radiant whilst embracing their natural features, rather than covering them up. I have volunteered for a couple of years now with *Look*

Good Feel Better, who are a charity that provide makeup classes for women who are undergoing cancer treatment. I love the power of makeup and I truly believe that putting some lippie on and doing your hair can make you feel better on the inside.

You may find that your skin changes during menopause; this is because your body stops making as much collagen. This along with dryness that you may experience due to hormonal changes can affect the way you apply your makeup. It's important to always start with moisturiser and allow this to soak in for a few minutes before starting your makeup. These skin changes can cause fine lines and sagging of the skin, and when makeup settles into fine lines it accentuates them. It is important to take care of your skin first as this has a huge impact on any makeup you wear.

When I have clients who are slightly older, I always use a beauty sponge (tip: use it damp not dry) as this allows you to blend the product into the skin. I start with a little and build. You want to make sure you use a nice sheer coverage foundation or a tinted moisturiser to avoid the product settling into any lines that you may have. I would avoid any products with the words 'matte', 'full coverage' and switch to 'dewy', 'buildable' and 'sheer'.

One of your main symptoms and possibly the most difficult as you may feel people notice, is redness from hot flushes. A great way to combat redness is to use a green concealer or primer. I have a very affordable green concealer from Collection 2000 and I like to put it under foundation and lightly blend it; this can help prevent any redness from appearing through your foundation throughout the day. Take time to get to know your changing skin and adapt to its new needs and you'll continue to glow throughout menopause.

Alcohol – Shane McClean

A note from Emma: My grandma always said "everything in moderation" and ladies, we all know drinking alcohol can sometimes bring on hot flushes, but there are occasions where you just have to say "feck it!"

Like it or not, alcohol plays a large part in a great many women's menopause, so rather than sweep it under the carpet, I thought it was best to address this head on. So I asked my friend Shane McClean, a famous mixologist from Barbados, to prepare something unique for all the menopausal women out there.

Shane is employed by, amongst others, the United Nations, to be the chief mixologist at their events, meaning he gets to travel the globe mixing cocktails in some of the fanciest locations on the planet.

When I explained to Shane what I was doing with this book, he kindly agreed to create a cocktail just for us. So here it is, go and grab the ingredients and give it a go!

And if you want to see the video of Shane mixing this, it's on my Facebook Group page.

The Menopausal Mix

Ingredients:
- One of two shots of white rum, gin or vodka
- Passion fruit juice
- 1 shot of cinnamon syrup
- Bottle of club soda
- Fresh basil
- Slice of lime & slice of orange
- Ice

Method:

Add the spirit of your choice to a tall glass with ice. Add a shot of cinnamon syrup and gently crush the fresh basil leaves before adding to the drink. Then, add passion fruit juice to fill the glass by one third, and top the glass up with club soda. Garnish with a slice of lemon and a slice of orange to finish.

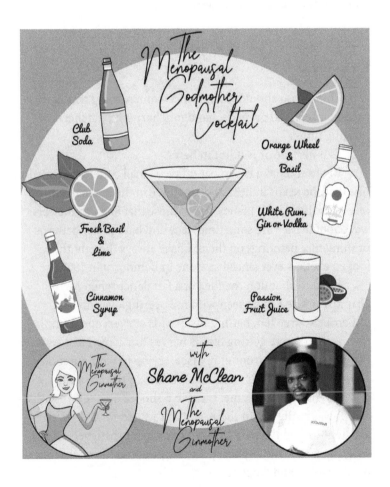

And of course, my Menopausal Godmothers chapter wouldn't be complete without some input from the lovely (and hilarious) Carol Wyer, who very kindly wrote the foreword for this book. Carol wrote *The Grumpy Menopause*, which was a bestseller and ended up with her being discussed on the Zoe Ball Breakfast Show on Radio 2! It has helped many women cope with menopause and encouraged them to do it with a smile on their face. Take it away, Carol!

H is for Hot Sweats, hula hoops, hair loss and humour– Carol Wyer

Things you should hide from a woman going through menopause: hand grenade, handgun, harpoon, hatchet, hunting knife.

"Is it just me or is it hot in here?"

My friend has a fan in her office, a small battery-operated one that she keeps in her handbag, three in the kitchen and one in the bedroom. I fancy one of those that Spanish dancers wave about. They are sometimes lacy and have pretty patterns or miniature paintings on them. I have always thought they looked exotic—ever since I saw one in Benidorm in 1977.

I had to abandon the idea of a fan dance when Mr Grumpy refused to be seen with me peering over my ludicrously large fan, batting my eyelids at everyone. I think the castanets were getting on his nerves too. Now I just wave my hands about in front of my face, trying to whir air about.

Yes, the dreaded hot flushes (flashes in the U.S.) can creep up on us at any time. I was in a shoe shop a few months ago. It was really hot in there, and as I waited for the young assistant to find the pair of shoes I fancied, I shrugged off my coat, my jacket and my scarf. The lady behind the counter saw me disrobing and laughed.

"At least you didn't do the same as me," she ventured, "I was out at dinner with friends and my husband last week and I suddenly felt a hot flush coming on. Of course, it was cold, being January, but I heated up like a furnace. I whipped off my jumper that I had put on. I wiped my face and thought that I'd got away with it, hoping no one had noticed I had just had a hot flush. My friends were sitting open-mouthed and my husband was aghast. I'd pulled off my blouse along with the jumper and I was sitting there in just my bra!"

Here's an explanation of what actually causes a hot flush, so at least you understand why you burn up. (I knew that "O" Level in Biology would come in useful one day.)

The hot flush is an alteration in thermal stability, which is maintained by the hypothalamus, a brain region located above the pituitary gland on the brain's floor. The hypothalamus operates the body's temperature regulation system. Oestrogen levels manipulate some functions of the hypothalamus. During menopause, as the ovaries produce less oestrogen, the hypothalamus senses and responds to the lower oestrogen levels by rapidly changing body temperature. The result may be a hot flush.[10]

You might want to consider some of the following for hot flushes: phytoestrogens, Black cohosh, Siberian rhubarb, acupuncture, hormone replacement therapy, or anti-depressants (SNRIs such as Effexor and Pristiq).

Chat to a medical person or someone who is qualified before embarking on a course of any homeopathic or herbal remedies—at least one study[11] has found that a combination homeopathic remedy can be useful in the treatment of hot flushes. This study found no adverse side effects from the treatment.

---

10 Source: http://www.fda.gov/fdac/features/1997/297_meno.html
11 http://www.ncbi.nlm.nih.gov/pubmed/22852580

I have found the cure for hot flushes.
Chocolate! Does it work? I don't know and
as long as I have chocolate, I don't care.

If we are going to get heated we may as well have a good reason to break out into a sweat. Taking up the hula hoop will make you feel about ten years old and will give you a terrific workout. It will allow you to display your youthful exuberance and once you've mastered the art again, you'll be able to showcase those hips. To add some extra sizzle, upgrade to a fire hoop!

Talking of sizzle, but of a different sort, I just discovered a rather unusual hobby—collecting handcuffs. At first, I thought this might be a tad bizarre, but now I think I can see the logic of it. Imagine the fun you could have locking your husband or children up in handcuffs and then claiming you have lost the key.

One of the most problematic parts of the menopause for me has been the migraine headaches. When you get a bad headache, you can feel awful about almost everything else. Hormonal imbalance during menopause may cause headaches. There are a variety of remedies but before you grab a box of aspirin, think about acupuncture. I admit that at times I would sooner be sticking pins in effigies of people I dislike rather than have someone sticking them in me; however, I should say that acupuncture has helped many women, especially those suffering from migraine headaches.

I also discovered Co-Q-10 thanks to a lovely lady, Chris Tryon, who I met in one of the Facebook menopause groups. It is good for your heart and can also alleviate headaches/migraines. The safest maximum dosage is 100 milligrams twice a day.

If you prefer to ride them out, take heart in the fact that once you are through the menopause, there is a high chance that your headaches will also disappear.

I feel it is my duty at this point, to remind you that sex also helps alleviate those nasty headaches. Research has shown[12] that the release of endorphins from sexual activity can reduce headache pain. It's much more fun than acupuncture and cheaper than a packet of headache pills. So next time you feel a headache coming on, grab your partner and treat them to a workout.

Do you remember that song by Peter Sellers, 'Goodness Gracious Me', in which Sophia Loren sings about palpitations? Whenever I get heart palpitations, I sing the lyrics of that song to myself. Guess what? It helps calm me down. If you have ever had heart palpitations, you will understand how frightening they can be. You fear the worst and wonder if a heart attack isn't imminent. I usually stick my leg out of bed, since it nearly always happens at night, to get contact with the floor, then sing to myself. Don't sing out loud or your other half will think you are completely mad. Try and sing it with appropriate accents too, for added amusement:

"A flush comes to my face. And my pulse begins to race. It goes boom boody-boom boody-boom boody-boom. Boody-boom boody-boom boody-boom-boom-boom."

I must bring herbal remedies to your attention in this section. I have had little personal experience of any herbal remedies, however, I discovered Jan Tucker who is passionate about the uses and benefits of herbs, with good reason, since she has used them to treat a variety of symptoms including bronchitis with great success. Herbs, and Ayurvedic herbs, also helped her sail through the menopause. Her website is most interesting. Again, I'll leave you to make up your own mind if you want to pursue this. Check her out at http://www.whitelotusliving.com/

---

12 http://www.redorbit.com/news/general/1112798056/sex-cures-headaches-030513/

One of the best ways to deal with all menopausal symptoms, apart from exercising and laughing, is to take up a hobby.

There are way too many hobbies to mention in this book but rather than looking at the traditional hobbies that women take up, why not consider attempting an adventurous activity like hiking, horseback riding, hot rodding, helicopter flying, hang gliding, hockey, or hunting?

There is also the rather unusual activity of hen racing. Yes, hen racing. You did read that correctly. Every year, hundreds of hens race against each other down a short course in Bonsall near Matlock, Derbyshire. Owners are not allowed to use anything other than verbal encouragement to help the hens complete the course. So, you get to meet like-minded hen owners, shout your head off and then go home and collect some eggs for tea. Sounds ideal to me.

Question: Who tells chicken jokes?
Answer: Comedihens.

There are a few menopausal symptoms that you might experience beginning with the letter H. I have talked about hot flushes and headaches but some women also suffer with hair loss. My research suggested that you should have your thyroid checked if you are losing hair, as it might not be due to hormone imbalance and falling levels of oestrogen. Unfortunately, thinning hair or loss of hair can make you feel dreadful about yourself. There are a number of treatments and hair-thickening shampoos available, but often a healthy balanced diet should help.

It is important to have a nutrient-rich diet, so don't embark on any weight loss diet programmes at this time and try not to endure too much stress in your life.

I found throwing a stress ball at Mr Grumpy worked well for me.

And a final note from me, Emma...

You've had some great advice from a range of specialists, all of whom were happy to share their knowledge and experience with you for this book. I'd like to personally thank each and every one of them.

From me, as a final note, as well as the top tips you've had in this chapter, I'd also like to recommend Music Therapy.

Did you know that listening to 5-10 songs a day can improve memory, strengthen your immune system and reduce depression risk by 80%? Sometimes listening to music can act as a distraction and changes your mood in a positive way. Perhaps you have a favourite song that gets you pumped up? Or maybe listening to a certain song helps you to escape. Whatever the reason, just listening to music can be a real "pick me up", especially when the day seems to be nagging at your heels.

WARNING: do not listen to Leonard Cohen, Bob Dylan or Joni Mitchell as they are likely to spiral you into deeper melancholy!

And finally, of course I am also going to recommend acupuncture! If you've never tried it, then go on, give it a go. What have you got to lose?

It's now time to move on to some other knowledgeable people – Three Wise Men who know exactly what it is like to live with a woman going through the menopause!

CHAPTER EIGHT

The Impact
(The Three Wise Men)

I t's all very well writing about the menopause and how it has affected me and thousands of women like me; but to do so in isolation, which many other menopause books do, is a mistake.

In most cases, there are other people involved: friends, family, children and especially partners. And in the research and reading I did prior to writing this book, it became clear that the ones without a say in this were the men.

Sure, they don't suffer the symptoms of menopause, but if they are close to you they are going through this every bit as much as you are.

When you wake in the middle of the night in a hot sweat and throw the covers off, they feel it. When you lose your temper over something insignificant, they feel it. And when you feel you can't cope and the walls are crashing in on you, they are the ones that are there for you.

So, to balance the scales a little bit, I felt it right to ask a few of them to contribute to this book.

I started by asking on Facebook and from that I had two

brave souls volunteer to write about their experience of going through the menopause with their wives. I also asked my husband and it is these Three Wise Men who have contributed the following.

Geoff's Story

Firstly, it's something blokes do talk about... well at least they did when I was first at work in the early 70s. I remember listening to the banter at tea breaks between the older guys and it was a subject that received some discussion. I gleaned at that early age when "she who must be obeyed" (at home anyway) was going through "the change", to "put up and shut up".

It might be different today, but back then building sites were pretty robust places to work and many of the older guys had served in WW2 – my gaffer had been a desert rat under Montgomery and fought in North Africa, Sicily and Italy. He didn't hold back when he had something to say.

Sharron's menopause journey started around four years ago. I guess I was oblivious to it to begin with. I had noticed that she was a bit more emotional than normal and her short fuse had grown shorter. But we had a pretty stressful house back then – me post stroke, a poorly son and Sharron trying to hold it all together. So it became tense at times – not really bad but short sharp words and bickering were pretty common.

Talk about it to your family and tell them what you are going through. They may not understand but at least they know how you are feeling.

SS

106

At first I put it down to circumstances and I didn't catch on until Sharron's periods started becoming irregular. Sharron went to the doctors to check that nothing untoward was going on and there wasn't. That's when the lightbulb came on and I realised what was happening. I decided then that the best way to support her was by not turning her emotional state – which was out of her control – into something that came between us. So I tried my very best to let it all wash over me and just be there for her. I guess the words "put up and shut up" were more apt than I realised and was probably the best advice a bloke could have – along with lots of hugs, reassurance and helping round the house.

Sharron has had all the normal menopause symptoms: sweats, change in diet etc. etc. But she's there now and we've both come out the other side better for it. We are both more tolerant and I realise that we just have to learn how to live with and accept that it's just a new chapter in our lives, much as I did after my stroke. I guess from my viewpoint, it wasn't really a biggie – it's just what you do when you love someone.

Tim's Story

I have had the misfortune of seeing the effects of the menopause on Sally twice! The first time was over a long period of years and I wasn't prepared for it in any way. The second time is most recently post hysterectomy, and this is far easier as it isn't as brutal for her either, and I was prepared for it too.

If I had any words of advice for men who are about to, or currently going through this with their wives/partners, I would say learn as much as you can about it and talk to your partner. Men are simple creatures compared to women and we are not taught anything about the menopause. We all know the jokes about hot flushes, but we have no idea what causes them or what our partners are experiencing. We can't understand why someone feeling hot makes them a nightmare to be around, with short tempers and what we see as "unreasonable behaviour".

I experienced days of rapid changes in temperament and snappy retorts to things I may have said, followed by fantastic days of a "normal" wife again. Only for this to change again because something minor has happened. This made me defensive and scared to say anything in case it unleashed the beast in Sally!

As well as the mental torment, there were obviously times when Sally felt unwell, not wanting to do things that a week ago she had been looking forward to. We had many an evening out cancelled because she didn't feel like going. Again, this caused resentment at times which changed the atmosphere in the house.

Sometimes this would recover quickly, others, it could take days. That is another thing that is hard to manage, never knowing how long one of these episodes would last. With hindsight, and it's really obvious when you have come out the other side, me learning more and having the patience to understand what she was going through would have eased the situation. At the time, though, this is not on the radar in any way as you have no real warning of its sudden impact – or at least I didn't. You also have to consider that there are often kids/teenagers around who are also going through life changes and this can exacerbate the tension and supercharge the already tense atmosphere.

Now, I'm an old hand at it and we talk about things far more – easier now there is just the two of us – but also we both have a far greater knowledge of what is happening and can adapt far more easily.

Jonathan's Story

I'm Jonathan, AKA 'The Anorak',[13] and in real life married to *The Menopausal Godmother*. And let me start by saying I really love my wife; always have, always will.

I wanted to get that out of the way first, so you can understand that what you read in this chapter is written out of love. In many ways, that sentence is as much for her as for you, the reader, as there are times when the demons of anxiety are battering away at her mind, when she wonders if I really do still love her. Of course I do, and hopefully the following will give some perspective on that.

When I was first asked to write something for this chapter of the book I wasn't overly keen. The writing bit wasn't a problem but a chapter of a book on a subject with which I was so closely involved? That's a real challenge. Seeing the wood for the trees is a skill I don't always possess, especially in matters of the heart.

Part of the issue is that I have to write about how the menopause has changed our relationship, but in reality, I really don't think that our relationship has changed at all. In my head it's the same now as it's always been, and we are both still in our 30s and 40s as we were when we first met.

So, accepting that whatever time I have left will be spent with my wife, the woman I fell in love with and married all those years ago, is something that I'm very happy with. Of course, it's not a problem as she's the woman I love and the woman I vowed to cherish and protect not just once, but twice.[14]

So, here we are at a point I still love her as much as I always did, but I'm not sure she always sees it the same way

---

13 Because I am a stamp collector, a Birder and I love reading.

14 We renewed our wedding vows in 2016 on our tenth wedding anniversary. See, I really am an old romantic at heart.

as she has on many occasions asked me if I still love her, and how can I possibly still love her?

This is where the menopause really affects her and us, and if you are reading this chapter, there's a chance you are going through this as well. I know that Emma suffers from periods of anxiety which, given what she has gone through with the cancer and mastectomy, is perfectly understandable.

She worries about her body, about how her reconstructed breast looks, her weight and body shape (which I still love by the way) and the toll that the menopause is having on her physically as well as mentally. And she has to carry all this round with her every day, and still function as a normal human being. She still works full time across three jobs: she's a director in two businesses and deals with palliative care and end of life cancer patients every week as an acupuncturist, listening to all their stories. It's a miracle she doesn't collapse under the weight of all this.

But she doesn't, she carries on. She goes to work and then comes home to me and our son, William. And we do try our best to be there for her. I do try to be supportive but even I can see that sometimes, no matter what I do, it's simply not enough.

There was a time when I wondered if it was the menopause or the operation which triggered the "change" in her, or both? Then I asked myself, does it make a difference?

The answer of course was "no"; whatever the trigger and however it has changed her, and by its nature, our relationship, this was and is still the woman I fell in love with.

But it's called the "change" for a reason and if our relationship and love for each other hasn't changed, what has?

The most obvious thing and the one that I'm sure will strike a chord with some of you, is that Emma occasionally has a shorter fuse. She was always a little bundle of energy and more than happy to fight her cause and that's part of what I fell in love with. But the thing that characterised the Emma I fell in love with is that she would pick up arms to fight a cause which made sense. She has a huge sense of what's right and wrong and hates to see injustice. She cares passionately about people and as a Parish Councillor for almost ten years did a huge amount for the people of her parish, finally delivering on some of the projects which had lain unfinished for years.

I could always see and make sense of the cause she was fighting. Even when it was something personal to us and I disagreed with her, I could always see her side of the argument.

Since the menopause, however, she sometimes sees injustice where I feel none exists. Sometimes it's the smallest thing that can set off an argument and there have been rare occasions when I'm not in the best frame of mind either, where we have gone from loving each other deeply to full blown argument in under ten seconds. I'm told that's not unusual with the menopause, but honestly, it doesn't make me feel much better about myself. I hate it when we argue and would far prefer everything was calmer.

I was told I should put some of these examples in the book, but the problem I have is, in honesty, I have to say that I can't remember a lot of these occasions. I have selective amnesia when it comes to remembering things like arguments and disagreements. When I'm prompted, things come to mind, which help and just to be able to write part of this chapter I had to ask Emma to help me recall times when things went awry, and we ended up disagreeing with each other!

As an example, on her birthday last year I really wanted to do something special for her and despite the fact that Emma hates surprises, I foolishly thought that organising a surprise for her was a good thing to do. I should have known better.

On the morning of her birthday she opened an envelope, inside which were details of a lovely spa day which I had planned and which we were going on that morning. Immediately as I told her we needed to be there by nine thirty, it went from being a lovely gesture to something else. Foolishly, I had completely forgotten that she didn't like surprises and so by giving her no time to prepare, I was rushing her, and by the time we left the house after whizzing around getting everything together, the mood was sour. This was not how I'd planned for her birthday treat to go!

In the car, halfway to the spa, she suddenly exclaimed that she had no swimming costume with her and of course, this was now my fault. If I hadn't surprised her and rushed her out of the house, we wouldn't be in this predicament. It had gone from big surprise, planned and delivered with love, to a frosty silence as we drove to the nearest Sainsbury's so she could buy a swimming costume.

Part of me just wanted to shout at her. How could she be so ungrateful? I'd spent so long planning this, asking friends for ideas, researching something we could do together and speaking to the venue to arrange the surprise, that to be sitting in that car, feeling as bad as I did, simply didn't make sense.

But at the back of my mind, I knew that she wasn't having a go at me. I knew that the reaction, whilst understandable in some respects, was not how she would normally react. When we first got together, something like this would have become one of our "couple's stories", something we could laugh about later.

Did it mean I loved her any less? Absolutely not. And sure enough, within an hour of being at the spa, in her lovely new swimming costume, we were both relaxed enough to return to normal and we spent a great day together.

How to deal with angry outbursts is probably something that will be personal to every couple. I know that my reaction is not always the best as frequently in these circumstances, I seem to escalate the situation rather than calm it.

I'm a logical type of person and often try the bloke thing of explaining why I think she's wrong. I'm telling you now, so you can benefit from my mistakes – this doesn't work. It never comes out as you expect it, and it's never received the way you might expect.

So, if trying to win the argument with logic is a non-starter, what does work? Well, there is one strategy which I have used which does work, to a point. When I asked Emma to remind me of things to put in this chapter, she recalled that sometimes when she's getting angry I have said to her, "I know it's not you, I'm going to walk away."

I'd actually forgotten about this (selective amnesia again) but the truth is that when I see the "menopause argument" arriving, I know it's not one I can win – ever. And the truth in the statement I make about walking away is I really do know it's not her. I know that it's out of character and she probably doesn't even want to fight.

I know as a man, accepting that we are wrong is hard, even when we are wrong, but this is one occasion when the best support you can give a woman going through the menopause is not to try and win the argument. Walking away prevents you from saying awful things to each other, as when arguments go beyond logic they tend to get personal, and in the heat of battle it's easy to say something you might regret later. If you really do love your wife or partner, walking away is sometimes the best thing to do, until you have both calmed down.

As part of the research for this segment, I read something that said 84% of women say menopause makes them feel negatively about themselves. It made me wonder, if that were 84% of men, would we know more about it? I guess we probably would and so I'm now firmly in the court which says we need to do more to help women who will inevitably go through this at some point in their lives.

It is essential not just for the support they need with the physical symptoms, but also for the mental symptoms. Women are more frequently judged and held to account by media pressure and stereotyping and, like it or not, this permeates into the societal "norms". So when a woman going through menopause finds she's putting on weight that she hadn't expected, despite the normal diets and exercise, and that her body shape is slowly changing away from the mid 30s body that she had become accustomed to, it must be hard to accept. Layer onto this a lowering of the libido and it's easy to understand why mentally she could feel unhappy with her looks, shape, weight and appearance.

And through all this, us men sit there and tell them that we love them. And we do. Ladies, I know it's hard to believe it, but we really do. We haven't changed (OK, so we have got older and fatter as well, but you might not see that the way we do) and we still want to be with the person we married.

I keep telling Emma that I made my mind up years ago and I stand by that. I did and I have, and nothing is going to change the view I hold that I want to grow old with her. And at some point, the menopause will be over, and we will both have changed. And I know, as we work though this, that we can stay together forever.

Emma's End Note

I would like to personally thank all the gentlemen for your frank and honest thoughts on what it is like to live with a loved one going through the menopause.

Honestly, it is so interesting to hear your side of things as most of the time we simply don't see this. Yes, we know you love us, but what I also took from your honest accounts is that even though it is us women going through the menopause, you go through it as well. Your journey is every bit as fraught as ours as you have to cope with us dealing with all our symptoms, and what's more, you have to do it with good grace. And for that we all thank you.

So, to all you gentlemen out there reading this and wondering what you can do if your wife or partner is going through the menopause, listen to these Three Wise Men:

- Take time to listen
- Understand it is not necessarily them who is speaking at that moment in time
- Try to learn a bit about the symptoms
- Keep the channels of communication open
- Know when to leave the room
- Keep loving her, no matter what.

And finally, to my Anorak, I love you too!

CHAPTER NINE

Letter From Emma

Dear Reader,

Many years ago, I remember thinking, "I would love to write a book" but the one doubt in my mind at that time was "What could I write about?" Fast forward oh so many years and the answer seemed to present itself. When I started this journey the book was supposed to be a straight account of how acupuncture works, with a particular focus on the work I had been doing with cancer patients suffering with hot sweats. Along the way, life happened (as you can tell from the previous chapters) and where I have ended up – where we have ended up – is a different place to that which I originally planned.

Well, after all that, here it is. And can I say a huge thank you from the bottom of my heart for not only buying this book but taking the time to read it. As I continue to go through the menopause myself, my one hope is that if this book has helped at least one other person cope with the debilitating symptoms, it has been worth all the time and effort. Perhaps this book has given you some ideas about new things that you could try, or at the very least, challenged your assumptions on the things that you can practically do if you are going through menopause.

It was in lockdown, brainstorming with my wonderful friend Gill Barham, that I came up with the name *The Menopausal Godmother*. Originally, the name was actually for her, but Gill said it just didn't suit her. Gill and I are menopausal specialists and work closely together as Godmothers. So, my vision for Gill, instead, became mine. On refection, I realised I had treated over a thousand women going through the menopause in my years as an acupuncturist, so when I came up with the name *The Menopausal Godmother*, I guess subconsciously I had decided that I actually deserved the badge.

I have written this book keeping in mind a friendly godmother that you can relate to, trust and someone who is independent to any of your friends and family. Because, quite frankly, you sometimes don't want to talk to them over and over again about how you are feeling. Not only will they tire quickly of hearing the same things from you over and over, but knowing you as well as they do it may be hard for them to understand and accept that you are struggling with the symptoms. A "godmother" therefore is someone you can talk to about your own journey, and whilst you don't need advice in the conventional sense of the word, you do need someone to listen and help you decide which path is best for you.

Us girls just want to get on with things, don't we? I hope that perhaps some of you recognise yourself in this book and know that you are not alone in this journey.

From inception, as soon as *The Menopausal Godmother* was given a name, it came to life and since then it has grown arms and legs. Creating this character has been huge amounts of fun and very exciting as well. The ideas have come thick and fast and each new idea, each new suggestion of what the "godmother" is, or could be, has sparked another round of inspiration and examination, culminating in the brand you see today. I wanted to say thank you to my wonderful stepdaughter, Gabriella, for coming up with the logo and helping me build this global brand. I love her and she is me.

So, we now have a website that has two discrete memberships: one for all the other Godmothers who are there to help ladies with the help, advice and a kindly ear; and the second for all you ladies going through the menopause. The website – menopausalgodmother.co.uk – and the membership is a safe, private space, for you to gain access to any of our godmothers' advice to help you. I'd long recognised the value of talking about what we are going through, in a safe environment, brought into sharp focus for me by the group sessions I ran at the hospice. I know that us women like to confide in each other and by facilitating an online safe space, this type of contact works for helping each other. Whilst there is no anonymity in the group – everyone uses their Facebook profile to join – the fact that you are amongst friends and away from anyone who might judge you makes this hugely effective as a way of coping.

Of course, It also has carefully selected products that you can buy and when it came to merchandise, it would have been all too easy to come up with a T-Shirt, mug and keyring with a clever slogan and offer these for sale like so many other websites, but I didn't want that. What I wanted was what I would like to see – thoughtful merchandise that both has form and function and is ideal for menopausal women. For example, I've examined hundreds of different tops before arriving at the range on the website today. I needed to find hard-wearing, good looking, breathable organic fabrics that would make a menopausal woman not just look good, but help with the problem of hot sweats. Similarly, the mugs needed to be china, not ceramic, as these conduct heat better. Some of the other products are "off the cuff", like the gin, which I knew would appeal to a number of women, and as soon as I found a supplier it seemed the right thing to do. Even the supplier for this was vetted and chosen because their gin removes all impurities at source and means you are less likely to end up with a headache the morning after. Of course, this depends on you enjoying it in moderation!

Seeing *The Menopausal Godmother* take shape has given me huge motivation and has been enormous fun. That reminds me, I had better mention Katie Webster, as she was the one who gave me a massive kick up the backside and is so supportive and funny when I say "It's going global, darling."

But actually, that is exactly where I see this brand going. Because it is an online space, it means that any member, anytime and anywhere in the world, can access the resources. On a laptop, table or mobile phone, as long as you can get online you are moments ways from help and support. And perhaps as it grows, I may have godmothers all over the world? Now there is an idea for another book…

So, finally, as *The Menopausal Godmother* I want to leave you with my last thoughts. My membership to the "cancer club" is one I cannot unsubscribe, but there it is – I am a member. I found that over the last few years I call this membership "Hotel California", simply because of the line in the song that goes:

"You can check out any time you like, but can never leave."

So, I wave my magic wand, and if I can't check out then I might as well be booked into the 'Presidential Suite' and sit at the bar drinking a crisp glass of top notch Sancerre. It's me moving on from fear and worry to acceptance and dealing with the situation.

The word "acceptance" means the action of consenting to receive or undertake something offered, a willingness to tolerate a difficult situation. Well, that kinda says it all. So, ladies, accept what happens to you along this journey of life. I cannot change the things that have happened to me, but I found my blend of techniques, products and help form my "survival kit" and I carry this along the way to help me. Hopefully, this book will form part of your own personal survival kit.

It is predicted by 2025 there will be over 1 billion (yes, 1 billion) women experiencing the menopause in the world, so if you would like to get in touch, join or help shape this global brand then please do so via any of our social media channels.

The "menopause club" is now only going to get bigger and I am aiming to reach and help as many women as possible with @menogodmum.

So, please follow me on Facebook, Twitter and Instagram; like, share, comment and help me to spread the word. Oh, and please don't forget to leave a review on whichever platform you buy this book. Individually, we are women going through the menopause; collectively we can be a force for good in this world. With your help, we can make a lasting difference.

And finally, live, love, laugh. With patience and good humour you can make your menopause no pause at all.

 x

CHAPTER TEN

Resources

I n writing this book and in my work life, I have done hundreds of hours of research and spoken to thousands of women going through the menopause. Whilst the wisdoms of individual women in this situation cannot be accessed online or in a manual, I hope I've been able to distil their messages into the chapters of this book.

Of course, there are plenty of other resources out there for women going through the menopause and I would encourage all of you to go on your own journey of discovery. You may just find the one thing that helps you more than anything else.

There are some resources that I used in the creation of this book and I wanted to list them here, along with the contact details of the people who contributed so willingly to chapters six and seven in this book, so you can further your reading and research and learn more about what is a critical period in your life.

Useful Online Resources

If you wanted to get in touch with any of the lovely people who contributed to Chapters six or seven in this book, here they are:

Naomi Gilmour –
https://www.naomigilmour.com/mindset-reframing-tools/

Dr Gill Barham –
www.drgillbarham.com **and** www.radiantmenopause.com

Gerard Lambe –
https://reflectclinic.co.uk/

Rosie Heaton –
http://www.puremindhypnotherapy.co.uk

Yifan Nairn –
https://atelier-5.co.uk/about/

Emma Wilson –
www.emmawilsonfitness.co.uk

Mindy Cowap –
www.mytimeforchange.co.uk

Sharron Roughton –
https://www.cheshirelasers.co.uk/sharronroughton.html

Steph Fox –
https://www.facebook.com/Steph-fox-mobile-Beautician-1566833976894404/

Toni Mackenzie –
https://www.innerdepths.co.uk

Paula and Nicola –
https://www.facebook.com/Thecuttingloungenorthwich/

Shane McClean –
https://www.instagram.com/mrshanemcclean/

Carol Wyer –
https://www.carolwyer.co.uk

Millennial Burnout –
https://www.instagram.com/millennialburnoutofficial/

Other Useful Resources:

Menopause Support – https://menopausesupport.co.uk
Menopause Doctor – https://www.menopausedoctor.co.uk

Useful Books

*Reading a book for 6 minutes a day can
reduce your stress levels by up to 68%*

- Haslam, P. (2019). *Make Yourself a little bit Famous.* SRA Books.
- Maher, E. (2020). *The Killing of Tracey Titmass.* Beaten Track.
- McLean, A. (2018). *Confessions of a Menopausal Woman.* Penguin.
- Mukherjee, A. (2021). *The Complete Guide to the Menopause.* Penguin.
- Newson, L.R. (2019). *Menopause.* Haynes.
- Pickles, S. (2016). *The Shock Factor.* Create Space Independent Publishing Platform.
- Powell, P. (2019). *50 Things I Wish I'd Told You.* Pavilion.
- Wyer, C.E. (2013). *Grumpy Old Menopause.* Safkhet Select.

Appendix

MYCaW[15] data: Acupuncture for Hot Flushes

Data collated independently by staff at St Luke's Hospice, Winsford. With grateful thanks to Wendy Wilson, Director of Care, for letting me publish this data.

Introduction

The acupuncturists at St. Luke's Hospice hold out-patient clinics at Winterley Grange on Wednesdays and at the Winsford site on Thursday afternoons. Patients were referred from breast care nurses, GP's and Breast Consultants, as well as internal referrals from the Hospice staff, working with patients who they felt might benefit from receiving some acupuncture.

Most appointments are on a one-to-one basis, but the service also provides group sessions for people suffering from (treatment/medication-induced) hot flushes. If availability allows, the acupuncturist who works on a Thursday also sees patients staying on the in-care unit and/or attending Day Hospice on that day.

MYCaW (Measure Yourself Concerns and Wellbeing)

The acupuncture service started using MYCaW in March 2014. Apart from the group sessions, the number of appointments a patient attends is determined by the acupuncturist, based primarily on their response to the treatment. Consequently, for group and one-to-one sessions, MYCaW forms are given to the participants on their first and last visits.

---

15 https://pubmed.ncbi.nlm.nih.gov/17352970/

Of the 36 patients that completed their MYCaW forms in 2015, the average number of sessions attended was 7.8 (range 5-16).

MYCaW – Completion Rates

Between March 2014 and 31ˢᵗ December 2015:
34 patients completed Part 1, but for the reasons below did not complete a Part 2:

- 3   died before was due to complete Part 2
- 6   were too poorly to carry on attending
- 4   people self-discharged themselves
- 19   did not attend their final session
- 2   Part 2 was not completed on their final visit.

In the same period, 60 MYCaWs (Parts 1 and 2) were completed. Some people said they only had one concern/problem, so only 47 completed scores were collected for "Concern/problem 2".

MYCaW – Numerical Results

For people attending the Acupuncture clinic, a statistically significant *improvement* was seen for all three of the self-scored questions.

This table shows the range of problems/concerns that respondents to the survey revealed, from hot sweats, pain and sleep problems to issues with body image and memory/cognition.

Break Down by Problems / Concerns	Part 1 Respondents	Problem 1	Problem 2	Part 2 Respondents
Hot Flushes / Sweats	57	48	9	41
Pain	34	17	17	17
Sleep Problems	21	5	16	14
Other Physical Concerns / Symptoms	16	9	7	9
Anxiety / Stress / Panic	10	5	5	5
Mood / Confidence / Coping / Control	6	1	5	5
Weakness Or Lack Of Energy (Fatigue)	7	3	4	4
Shortness Of Breath	5	3	2	3
Body Image	4	0	4	3
Other Medical Conditions	3	2	1	2
No Problems	2	0	2	2
Poor Mobility	1	0	1	1
Family & Relationships	1	1	1	1
Memory / Cognition	1	0	1	0
Poor Mobility	1	0	1	1
Family & Relationships	1	1	1	1
Memory / Cognition	1	0	1	0

Part 1 survey asked the respondents to prioritise their main symptom (Problem 1) and the second biggest symptom (Problem 2). The Part 2 survey at the end of the clinical study asked which symptoms were still an issue for the respondent.

MYCaW Score

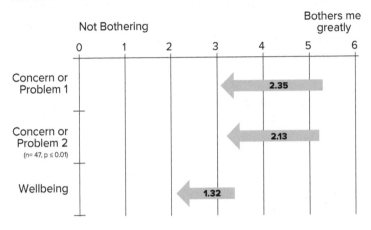

Figure – Change in MYCaW Score for pooled Acupuncture data, paired t-test
(Where the arrow indicates the direction of change, shows an improvement from Part 1 score [square end] to Part 2 score [pointed end] and colour green = statistically significant).

On the 7-point scale, where 6 = "Bothers me greatly" and 0 = "Not bothering me at all", the largest change (-2.35) was from 5.43 to 3.08 for "Concern or Problem 1" (n = 60, p ≤ 0.01). Similarly, the average reduction in how much "Concern or Problem 2" was bothering them was -2.13 (from 5.34 to 3.21).

The question asking *"How would you rate your general feeling of wellbeing now?"* is also scored on a 7-point scale, where 6 = "As bad as it could be" and 0 = "As good as it could be". Though the improvement in wellbeing was smaller, from 3.41 to 2.09, it was also statistically significant (n = 58, p ≤ 0.01).

Results were further analysed by pooling the completed data from "Concern or Problem 1" and "2", then grouping the responses by theme. The most common themes were:

	(Number)
Hot flushes / sweats	*(41)*
Pain	*(17)*
Sleep problems	*(14)*
Other physical concerns / symptoms (e.g. headaches, arthritis)	*(9)*

All themes showed an improvement, i.e. there was an average decrease in how much they were bothering those people. Paired t-tests were used again to explore the results, but as sample sizes smaller than 15 considered too small for statistical analysis only two Concerns were tested.

MYCaW Score

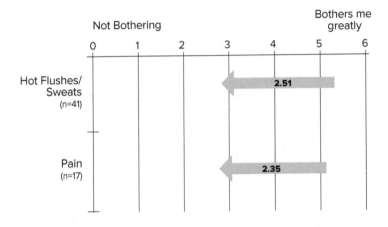

Figure – Change in MYCaW Score for most reported Concerns or Problems in Acupuncture Clinic, sorted by amount of change, paired t-test
(Where the arrow indicates the direction of change, shows an improvement from Part 1 score [square end] to Part 2 score [pointed end] and colour green = statistically significant).

Of the completed MYCaW forms, 68.3% of people said one of their "Concerns or Problems" was "Hot flushes and/ or sweats". This was the single most-reported theme of any of the Hospice services described in this report, and showed a statistically significant improvement from 5.32 (where 6 = "Bothers me greatly") to 2.81, a change of -2.51. Similarly, "Pain" saw statistically significant improvement from 5.12 to 2.77 (a change of -2.35).

MYCaW – Written Comments

Part 2 of the validated MYCaW forms asks:

WHAT HAS BEEN MOST IMPORTANT FOR YOU?

Reflecting on your time at the **Acupuncture Clinic** at St. Luke's Hospice, what were the most important aspects for you?

(write overleaf if you need more space)

Of the 60 completed forms, 59 comments were left in this box. As with the comments written by Day Hospice patients, a simple word count method was used to analyse the responses. All of the responses were assessed in this way and the features of the Acupuncture Clinic that were most frequently mentioned as being most important to attendees were:

	(Number)
Improvement in hot flushes / sweats	*(17)*
Acupuncturist	*(13)*
Being able to relax / feel at ease	*(12)*
Company / group / making new friends	*(11)*
Increased confidence / well-being / feeling more positive	(10)
Improved sleep	(8)
Talking / chatting / being listened to	(7)

"What has been most important for you?"

Actual responses included:

"(The acupuncturist)and the group therapy has been great. I feel a lot better than before. Thank you and made new friends! ☺"

"A certain amount of improvement in my general well being, and a positive outlook have developed. I found (acupuncturist) to be very knowledgeable, understanding and a pleasure to be with."

"Being offered help, having time to find some comfort and support to help me as a person as well as the symptoms. Someone who is able to listen and then help the body and mind to open up the healing itself. Looking back, there has been a definite improvement in the trend of the symptoms, which makes an important difference to well-being."

"Being explained how acupuncture works has helped. The fact that the treatment has been wonderful has been important."

"Dedicated 'me time'. Time and opportunity to talk to others in a similar situation."

"The expertise and time spent in helping me reduce my hot sweats and sleeplessness has been invaluable. I now sleep much better and my hot sweats are manageable."

"Excellent service. (The acupuncturist) offers first class. Acupuncture – helped my hot flushes."

"To help my major sweats as they had become unbearable and I was unable to sleep properly as well and (the acupuncturist) has helped me greatly."

"It has been a lovely experience, very relaxing and lovely making new friends. (Acupuncturist) has helped greatly with the sleeping and hot flushes they are now a lot better on the whole and the relaxation techniques have also helped. Thank you so much for a really lovely time."

"Notable beneficial results, excellent therapist."

"Found that it has helped me and built self-esteem back again. Sleeping much better."

"Friendly staff. Excellent knowledge and support."

There's not enough space in this book for me to publish the entire raw data set, but if anyone needs it, please do get in touch with me and I'll be happy to share it with you.

About Emma

Emma was born and bred in Northern Ireland in 1969 at the start of the 'Troubles'. She moved to Cheshire in 1985 and now resides in Northwich with her husband, Jonathan, and William, their teenage son. Gabriella and Marcus, the older children, have flown the nest.

Emma started her career as a welder – yes, you read correctly. I guess from a very early age Emma has always wanted to fix things, perhaps even to fix people too. In case you wanted to ask, she preferred electric arc welding to Oxyacetylene.

Emma absolutely loves music; in fact, this was her favourite and most studied subject at school. She mainly played the viola but she loved to sing, drum and play the recorder. Her first love of music (and still is) is classical music. Emma also still likes to sing and dance around the house, mostly when she has had a few wines.

Emma is loyal, loving and has a big heart, but do not abuse her trust because as soon as you cross that line there is no going back. I guess that is the 'Norn Irish' in her.

Her jobs to date are: Welder, Hairdresser, Receptionist, Sales Manager and now she is a Director for Aqueous Digital with her husband, Jonathan, and of course she runs the Acupuncture That Works Clinic.

This is Emma's debut book on how acupuncture can help you in menopause. She created the *Menopausal Godmother* online space in a private group on Facebook, with other Godmothers advising on matters such as fitness, nutrition, and hypnotherapy. Whilst she knows her own field, she got the help of other specialists in their fields to give factual, honest, helpful advice to ladies going through the menopause.

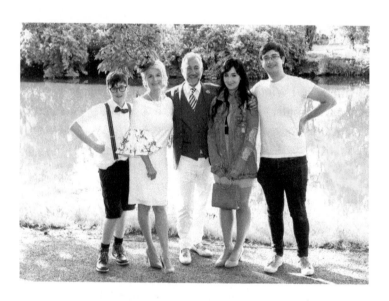

Acknowledgements

Firstly I have to thank my Grandfather William 'Papa Bill' for believing in me when others didn't. You made me be the person I am today. Whilst you passed away when I was only nine, you were the biggest positive influence in my life. Miss you still today, 42 years on, Papa.

To Jonathan, aka my Anorak, my forever soulmate, my husband. I am so in love with you and always will be. Thank you for taking our marriage vows so seriously and boy, haven't we done them all! I really don't know if I would be here without you, thank you.

To all my children: William, Gabriella and Marcus. You are all my favourites(!) and no trademark was needed. But, a little special thank you to Gabriella for creating The *Menopausal Godmother* book cover and logo.

To all my dearest friends, but in particular to Debbie, Karen and Fanta (Chris) who are there for me always, thank you.

To James Harvey, my oncology Breast Consultant, thank you for being the best of the best and I will always support your ongoing charity work for Prevent Breast Cancer.

To St Luke's Hospice for agreeing to let me use the data to show how acupuncture works. Some of the proceeds of this book will be given annually to you. Thank you.

To all my other Godmothers who helped me with factual advice for ladies going through the menopause. Thank you. A special thank you to Dr Gill Barham for mutually brainstorming our ideas of menopause support.

To Katie, Business Coach who gave me quite a large kick up the backside and got this whole thing rolling. Thank you.

To Sian, my book mentor, thank you for believing in me and holding my hand month by month on writing this book.

To Andrew Collier, for making me look wonderful whenever you photograph me, and for the family picture in this book.

Thank you to Tanya Bäck for making my book come alive with your design.

Thanks to Aga Mortlock for the picture on the back cover and all my branding photography.

Lastly but no means least, to all my wonderful patients over the last nine years who made the *Guy Protocol* happen. Thank you.

Lightning Source UK Ltd.
Milton Keynes UK
UKHW022054090421
381747UK00005B/40